AURAL REHABILITATION
FOR THE ELDERLY

The Symposium was sponsored by the Division of Communication Disorders and the Center for Studies on Aging, North Texas State University, and held in the University Union, October 12–14, 1978. Partial support was granted by the Department of Human Resources with the Moody Foundation and the Governor's Committee on Aging.

Symposium Director
Miriam A. Henoch, Ph.D.

AURAL REHABILITATION
FOR THE ELDERLY—

EDITED BY *Miriam A. Henoch, Ph.D.*

Assistant Professor and
Coordinator of Audiology
Department of Speech Communication and Drama
North Texas State University
Denton, Texas

GRUNE & STRATTON, INC.
A Subsidiary of Harcourt Brace Jovanovich, Inc.
New York   *San Francisco*   *London*

Grune & Stratton, Inc.
111 Fifth Avenue
New York, New York 10003

Distributed in the United Kingdom by
Academic Press, Inc. (London) Ltd.
24/28 Oval Road, London NW 1

Library of Congress Catalog Number 79-13158
International Standard Book Number 0-8089-1186-4
Printed in the United States of America

Contents

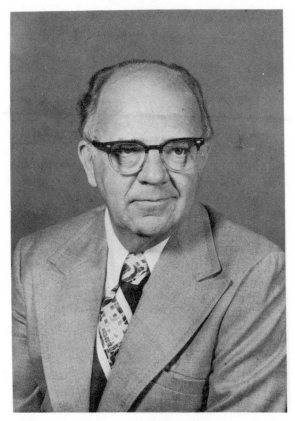

John H. Gaeth, Ph.D.
1913–1978

John H. Gaeth was chosen to present the keynote address at the Symposium on Aural Rehabilitation for the Elderly because he was not only a former teacher but a good friend as well. He was a logical choice because of his many years of experience in all aspects of aural rehabilitation.

On October 11, 1978, Dr. Gaeth died while on his way to attend the symposium. The loss was felt deeply by all who knew him, for he had given so much of himself to the profession he loved. This book is dedicated to his memory . . . the teacher, the friend.

Acknowledgments

The symposium and the subsequent publication of the proceedings could not have become reality without the time and efforts of a great many people.

I wish to thank the faculty and students of the Division of Communication Disorders at North Texas State University for their support and encouragement before and during the symposium. I especially want to thank Dr. Hiram Friedsam, co-director of the Center for Studies on Aging, whose initial efforts and support enabled us to obtain funding for the symposium.

I appreciate the hard work of Marian Benson and Pauline Peverly of the Center for Community Services, who took care of all the local arrangements.

Thanks are also due Mary Carolyn Yates and Beth Ryan for getting the manuscript ready for publication.

I am especially grateful to the Department of Human Resources with the Moody Foundation and the Governor's Committee on Aging, Texas, for their respective grants in partial support of the symposium.

A very personal thanks is due Irv Deshayes of the University of Nebraska, who very graciously agreed to present the keynote address of John Gaeth.

Finally, I wish to thank the guest faculty and the participants for making the symposium a highly successful interchange of ideas in the area of rehabilitative audiology for the elderly.

MAH

Participants

Jerome G. Alpiner, Ph.D.
Department of Communicative
    Disorders
The University of Mississippi
University, Mississippi

Carl A. Binnie, Ph.D.
Department of Audiology and
    Speech Sciences
Purdue University
West Lafayette, Indiana

John C. Cooper, Ph.D.
Division of Otorhinolaryngology
The University of Texas Health
    Science Center at San Antonio
San Antonio, Texas

John H. Gaeth, Ph.D.
Department of Audiology
Wayne State University
Detroit, Michigan

Dean C. Garstecki, Ph.D.
Northwestern University
Evanston, Illinois

Miriam A. Henoch, Ph.D.
Department of Speech
    Communication and Drama
Division of Communication
    Disorders
North Texas State University
Denton, Texas

Harriet Kaplan, Ph.D.
Galludet College
Washington, D.C.

Roger E. Kasten, Ph.D.
Department of Logopedics
Wichita State University
Wichita, Kansas

Robert L. McCroskey, Ph.D.
Department of Logopedics
Wichita State University
Wichita, Kansas

Brian Scott, Ph.D.
Scott Instruments
815 N. Elm
Denton, Texas

Herbert Shore, Ed.D.
Golden Acres
2525 Centerville
Dallas, Texas

AURAL REHABILITATION
FOR THE ELDERLY

Chapter 1

Keynote Address:
A History of Aural Rehabilitation[1]

JOHN H. GAETH, PH. D.

Clearly Aural Rehabilitation, as we know it today, began with the four retraining centers in World War II. The individuals who worked there were obviously satisfied with the results they had obtained for they set about to establish centers to provide similar services for civilians who were hearing impaired. The men and women who had been drafted and commissioned to set up programs for the hearing casualties of the war were the ones who set up the Hearing Clinics and changed Speech Clinics to Speech and Hearing Clinics beginning in 1946.

Originally, I had intended to summarize briefly the programs and the procedures in the Aural Rehabilitation Centers of World War II and then to lament about what little progress we have made in the past 35 years. As I looked for written material to support my memory, I found the notes from a Symposium which Carhart organized for the Summer School program at Northwestern University in 1946. I read the material, and I realized much of it had never been put into writing and probably never would. There was an impressive list of speakers for the Symposium and they spoke of experiences just past. While reading these notes I decided to summarize the materials of three of the lecturers most relevant to our topic here. First, Dr. Norton Canfield, a colonel in the Army, an otolaryngologist, and Associate Professor at Yale Medical School, was responsible primarily for setting up the aural rehabilitation centers in the army at Deshon General Hospital at Butler Pennsylvania, at Borden General Hospital at Chickasha, Oklahoma, and at Hoff General Hospital in Santa Barbara. Second, Dr. Francis L. Lederer,

---

[1]Dr. Gaeth's manuscript is printed here almost entirely as he wrote it. He had not finished editing the manuscript before his death and the Editor has chosen not to take liberties with the unedited portion of his manuscript.

captain in the Navy, Professor of Otolaryngology and Head,
Department of Otolaryngology, Medical College, University of
Illinois, had been responsible for the program at the Philadelphia Naval Hospital. Third, Dr. Raymond Carhart, acoustic
physicist at Deshon General Hospital, major in the Army, and
associate professor of speech, Northwestern University, wrote
most extensively on clinical procedures in audiology. These
three men had great influence on the programs developed by
the military forces and even greater impact on the subsequent
programs for civilians. Canfield was influential in the
development of the Veteran Administration programs. Lederer,
as head of the Illinois Eye and Ear Infirmary, developed one
of the more broadly based residency training programs in ENT
and one of the best service programs for hearing impaired
children and adults. Although Bunch had started the hearing
program at Northwestern University, Carhart built it into an
outstanding educational/clinical program out of which came
many outstanding audiologists. The material I am summarizing
here mostly comes unedited from the notes I took in the
Symposium Carhart organized for the six weeks summer session
at Northwestern University in 1946. The notes from Canfield
and Lederer had been transformed into typewritten copy, but
the notes from Carhart's lectures are still in the original
handwritten form.

Canfield called his lecture, "Battle Induced Hearing
Loss" and included under this label loss of hearing acuity
during war whether partial or complete, functional or
organic. He felt that sounds have different meaning during
wars and are probably far more important to self-preserva-
tion. For example, unilateral hearing is really not a great
civilian handicap but can be a big one during battle.

He was critical of the hearing tests used as part of
the induction examinations. A subcommittee on Otolaryngology
had been organized and then dissolved and then organized and
dissolved again without being able to make a real contribution. In spite of recommendations of the above groups, the
hearing tests used in the Induction Centers for World War II
were first the voice test and later the whisper test. Both
were inadequate and objective evidence with the decibel meter
indicated that with many testers the voice intensity was
greater at 15 feet than at 5 feet. This was probably due to
the fact that by reflex the voice is increased as the distance is increased and the tester is likely to be completely
unaware of the fact. As the result of the testing procedures, the army and the navy took a great many men with hearing losses. Of these, three to four thousand cases of
civilian deafness eventually appeared in the rehabilitation

centers. Canfield did not recommend that all men with hearing losses necessarily be kept out of the army but the fact of the hearing loss should have been considered in their placement; such individuals may do better than normal in noisy backgrounds or in airplanes.

The situation he described in the European theater was interesting. Because of the shortage of men and the difficulties of transportation across the Atlantic, orders were given to keep all men on service who could possibly be used. One group of 108 men in Europe were all fitted with Western Electric Aids which had been shipped over and later 400 Zenith Aids were sent over and issued. In general, the results were satisfactory. About 300 men were kept on duty because of these aids, and 75% of the 300 expressed satisfaction with their hearing aids. He said that he could not get an accurate picture of how soon after their injury these individuals were able to tolerate a hearing aid because of the military method of handling cases but still he thought that hearing aids should be a part of supply at all fronts.

Canfield mentioned again the differences between a unilateral hearing loss in civilian life and in war service. He felt the perception of the direction of sounds was very important, and a man with a unilateral loss might move in the wrong direction or lead his men in the wrong direction. Furthermore, if the good ear were damaged, the man would no longer be of service. He noted that "hearing traumas" were treated slowly, since the men were always side-tracked for flesh wounds.

He stated that an ear protector, "Ear Wart", a neophrene plug was developed at the Psycho-Acoustic Laboratory at Harvard but it reached the men late in the war and those who wore it said that it was uncomfortable. He thought the men should wear individually molded earplugs, and cited an instance where a dental officer dropped casualties from three percent to nearly zero through issuance of custom plugs.

Canfield devoted a portion of his lecture to the causes of deafness during the war. He discussed increased accidents, but my notes are incomplete here. He thought it would be some time before we could be sure of the degree of losses among the flyers, but he was optimistic that there would not be too much loss from normal or beyond previous loss, for the reason that the headphones worn provided protection from the noise. Frequently hearing loss was not noted until other wounds were treated and until the person was up and around. There was then a period of waiting for further assignment and frequently further recovery. This

left the question unanswered as to whether the defect was
organic or functional.

During battle, injury may be permanent if there was
actual destruction to the otic capsule or temporary if the
missile came near, in which case the loss may be temporarily
organic and later functional. There was no way of knowing
the number who temporarily lost hearing. The rule was that
if there was not recovery in three days the individual was
sent back from the front. He believed that entirely too many
hearing aids were issued.

There were many cases of injuries to the tympanic
membranes. Of these 17% healed in a month and 5% had acute
otitis media. In most cases where individuals with ruptured
membranes were tested, the hearing was found to improve after
healing. (He did not state whether the measured loss which
improved was sensory or conductive.) He did state that one
of the big difficulties with the research on the handling of
cases was the fact that there was no good induction test results to serve as frames of reference.

For rehabilitation there must be a convalescent period of from six to eight weeks during which time individuals
are grouped and treated according to hearing loss and
intellectual level. The level program should include acoustic training, speech correction, lip reading, adjustment to
a hearing aid, and psychiatric work to eliminate psychogenic
hearing losses. For this narco-synthesis was used and found
to be quite effective. He felt that there was a good possibility that 10% of the hearing loss was psychogenic and
further that there was no basis for knowing how much temporary acoustic trauma was due to psychogenic causes.

Finally, I record, as his closing remarks, the fact
that there was probably a significant amount of psychogenic
hearing loss in the civilian population and that a pure tone
audiometric test is of no use in diagnosing psychogenic hearing losses.

Dr. Lederer's lecture was entitled, "Adult Hearing
Problems on the Basis of Military Experience". He began by
stating that for conservation of hearing there needs to be a
coordinated program, which includes: otologists, psychologists, speech reading, speech correction, hearing tests,
prosthetics, counselors, physical education, vocational rehabilitation, etc. Rehabilitation of the hard of hearing is
primarily a nonmedical problem, but he felt best progress
came with a coordination of medical and nonmedical groups.

The navy program was called physical and psychosocial
therapy and the basic philosophy was that each staff person
should be conversant with the various areas listed above.

Service personnel were admitted if they had a loss of 30 dB
or more in the better ear. He stated that the speech reception test was a better threshold measure than a pure tone
test.

As far as the navy program was concerned, he offered
the following information on the patients served: (a) 40%
of the cases were hard of hearing before entering service
(He felt that the otologists had fallen down here); (b) 20%
were chronic progressive (mainly otosclerosis but some otitis
media); (c) 15% were perceptive (sensori-neural); and (d) 26%
were due to heavy gun fire, etc. On heavy firing, the unexpected salvoes were the most damaging and, of the naval
guns, the three- and five-inch were the worst. They also
found a few cases of quinine deafness.

He had little faith in the surveys that were being
reported: "Statistics are like a lamp post for a drunk--a
form of support but little illumination". His guess was
that there would be a quarter of a million men coming out of
the war with hearing impairments. He suspected that deafness
from heavy fire is a gradual degeneration with initial recovery, and cases may turn up again later in two, four, or
even eight years.

He spent considerable time talking about rehabilitation. At the outset the individual is given a picture of
what the program is and what its limitations are (If a
bastard before, rehabilitation will not change you). The
centralization of the focus of the navy program was on the
individual to give him the tools to live in a highly specialized hearing world. Each individual should be educated in
the problem and its solution.

The program should offer new abilities and skills.
On the positive side, offer speechreading, sound discrimination, hearing aids, etc., while on the negative side, need to
nullify neurotic tendencies.

Lederer did not think we could have a "Psychology of
the Hard of Hearing". It is true that there are types of
hearing impaired, but that is because we have types of
people. Pigeon-holing them is all right but you need to know
what you are going to do with the categories. Behavioral
typing would be simple if the loss had been an arm or a leg,
but a hearing loss is significant in terms of the total
personality. You must get the person to feel relatively
normal. He felt that private physicians wrongly hold out too
much hope to patients and that they needed a good sound
mental hygiene course instead which lays the cards on the
table and gives help on how to cope. He is now trying

gradually to train otologists in a new and better outlook.
He offered the following terse comments;

1. Audiometry must be carefully done on an instrument that
    is properly calibrated. Audiogram does not diagnose--
    you need a total picture for diagnosis.

2. Speech reception is a very important test, especially
    in noise.

3. Medical social workers will one day replace secretaries
    in physicians' offices. This would be a good move; they
    can serve as guidance counselors for the patient.

4. The psychologist serves as a personal father and con-
    fessor, very important in the recovery program.

5. Rehabilitation takes from four to eight weeks and is
    really a basic training course.

6. They classified their patients as Marginal, if 30-40 dB;
    Moderate, if 40-70 dB; and Severe if over 70 dB.

7. He does not think much of Ear Defenders at present.

8. The ones who suffered the hearing losses were the ones
    who had ear diseases; this fact should be taken into
    consideration in an induction procedure.

9. There were many cases of what he called "Situation Deaf-
    ness". The individual was exposed to a loud blast, found
    himself with a hearing loss, was finally shipped back to
    the States, but then noticed that his hearing was getting
    better on the way back. The individual became confused
    and did not understand what had happened. If he were to
    report what had happened, he might be accused of faking
    the hearing loss. He is now scheduled for return to the
    States, but, if he reports his improved hearing, he will
    likely be sent back to the mud at the front. The
    obvious solution is to go on pretending the hearing loss.

    Lederer did not think that this was true malingering and
    guessed the same condition could occur in industry, in
    which there was a loss when the legal action was started;
    then the hearing improves, but he cannot back out, so the
    case goes on. The way hearing is tested, the individual
    learns certain responses that help him to maintain the

picture. In this connection Lederer did not believe the navy had nearly the 15% malingerers reported in the army.

Lederer felt that each large community should have a clinic equipped to handle the total hearing diagnostic and rehabilitation program. He did not believe in specialized partial clinics which run the patients here and there. In a population of one million, about eight clinics are needed to handle the twenty thousand hard-of-hearing individuals. For communities which are too small to warrant a clinic, and for rural areas, he recommended a mobile clinic including--as far as possible--the same personnel and equipment that station-ary clinics would have.

My notes record that Lederer made very casual refer-ence to an article which was to appear, or had appeared, in the May *Archives of Otolaryngology*. That article was not on our reading lists for the Symposium, and I cannot remember anyone reviewing the article nor seeing it on any lists of references. After having transformed my notes into this presentation, I set out to locate his reference. To my sur-prise, it contained a 32-page article by Lederer and Hardy on the navy program. Much of it seemed to me to have rele-vance for us today. I then did a search of the references in the current books on aural rehabilitation: Alpiner, Oyer and Frankmann, and Sanders. The article is not mentioned in any of the three. However, the first edition of Hearing and Deafness contains a chapter by Canfield on Military Aural Rehabilitation, and the article is listed as a reference for that chapter.

The article by Lederer and Hardy was long enough that it contains several things that Lederer did not cover in his lecture. It states that the service experience with the re-conditioning and reconstitution of the hard of hearing as distinguished from the congenitally deaf furnishes a pattern and methods that can be translated efficiently into civilian needs under the leadership of American otologists. The goal of rehabilitation had been defined by Admiral McIntire as "all activities and services which may be required to supple-ment the ordinary or usually therapeutic procedures in order to achieve maximum adjustment of the individual patient . . . with the least possible handicap from his disability". The fundamental idea of such a program is its centralization in the rehabilitee's personality. The goal becomes the recon-stitution of the total person. There are at least three principal elements which characterize this approach to the rehabilitee's problems:

1. A man is more important than his ears. Specialists in
    hearing and speech proceed in the belief that they are
    under obligation to treat the total personality.

2. Recognition of the need to arrest deteriorating charac-
    teristics and to do everything possible to help restore
    the subject's complete existence; the rehabilitee must
    learn to become, not a handicapped person who travels
    alone, dependent and frustrated, but a person who wears
    a hearing aid, who is in communication with his fellows
    and who is as capable of economic and social efficiency
    within the limits of his potentialities as any other man.

3. There is the need to help an aural rehabilitee expand
    certain of his capabilities in order that he may compen-
    sate for a hearing loss in complex socioeconomic
    existence.

    Lederer and Hardy state that a program which is
patient centered must undertake two essential steps.

    The first is positive: the development of new abilities
    and skills, new tools to achieve efficient and success-
    ful behavior and adjustment. As positive therapy, mod-
    erate proficiency in speechreading, training in sound
    discrimination and supervised use of a hearing aid are
    fundamental elements of the patient's equipment for
    normal behavior.

    The second is negative: the understanding and nullifi-
    cation of the adverse effects that are inevitable by-
    products of any serious interference with communicative
    habits. The rehabilitee must learn new ways of getting
    along in a world that is dependent on communication.
    If he wears a hearing aid, he must learn to think and
    act like a person who wears a hearing aid, not like a
    person who is perfectly normal but cannot hear well.
    He must prepare himself to meet the thoughtless attempts
    of others to communicate with him.

    The staff at the Naval Hospital found the importance
of group therapy could hardly be overemphasized. From arri-
val until discharge the individuals met in groups where they
had or developed common interests. They met in groups with a
psychologist for mental hygiene, with the otologist for lectures and discussions of the hearing mechanism and

pathologies of the ear; they met for generalized discussions
of their problems, and later to discuss hearing aids and
their care.

The reeducational program was planned for from four
to six weeks with classes in speechreading and auditory
training scheduled five days a week. The speechreading program was built around the Jena method. This system utilizes:

A close correlation among speech, speechreading, and
auditory training of residual hearing. Its fundamental
precept is that the kinesthetic, or "feeling" form of
communication, is the only form that is complete for
everybody.

The patient spends hours talking simultaneously with
the instructor, while he sees, feels, and hears the
general pattern of expression. Then, in an effort to
recall all the sensations of the pattern when he spoke
it aloud, he watches the instructor while the same material is repeated. The next step is silent practice with
the instructor, who preferably addresses the group from
a position behind a soundproofed glass partition.

The scope of the speechreading program is shown in
Figure 1. The training was given to small groups, six to
ten, with similar natural ability. Groups did not stay the
same, and each group was assigned to a new instructor each
week.

As shown in Figure 2, auditory training was divided
into four main parts: (a) adjustment to amplified sound,
(b) learning to use the hearing aid in life situations, (c)
knowledge of functional hearing, and (d) consideration of
future problems. They used a group aid, with a single earphone in preparation for the monaural body aid, to give practice in listening to amplified speech. The patients listened
through the earphone and through a speaker to vocal and
instrumental music, speech and sound effects, in quiet and in
noise. In their experience, these early experiences with the
group aid made adjustment to the individual aid much easier
for the patients.

Apparently all four centers felt that speech training
and correction was an important part of the rehabilitation
program. At the naval center, the patients were given daily
exercises in articulation and discrimination of sound.
Lederer and Hardy state:

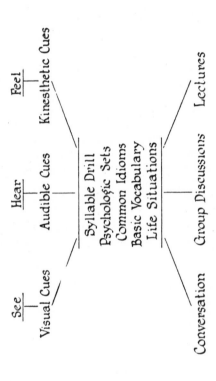

FIG. 1. *Schematic outline of the course in speech reading of the Speech and Hearing Rehabilitation Unit, United States Naval Hospital, Philadelphia.*

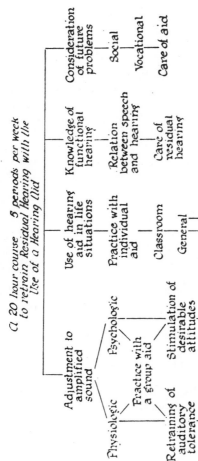

AUDITORY TRAINING

A 20 hour course — 5 periods per week
to retrain Residual Hearing with the
Use of a Hearing Aid

Adjustment to amplified sound
- Physiologic
  - Retraining of auditory tolerance
  - Retraining of auditory intelligibility
- Psychologic
  - Practice with a group aid
  - Stimulation of desirable attitudes
    - Toward hearing loss
    - Toward use of aid

Use of hearing aid in life situations
- Practice with individual aid
  - Classroom
  - General
    - Social
    - Economic

Knowledge of functional hearing
- Relation between speech and hearing
- Care of residual hearing

Consideration of future problems
- Social
- Vocational
- Care of aid

FIG. 2. Schematic outline of the course in auditory training of the Speech and Hearing Rehabilitation Unit, United States Naval Hospital, Philadelphia.

Special attention is paid to the patients' articulatory habits in an effort to tone up their speech
patterns. The goal of this phase of the rehabilitation effort is not to put the emphasis on any special
pattern of speech but to foster clear serviceable
speech and to stress the relation between speech and
hearing. The patients must learn discrimination in
the production of their own speech and know how to
guard against the deterioration of speech . . .

The article reports on a questionnaire sent to 1,172
former patients. At the time of writing, 508 had been returned and 490 were used for a summary. They found:

1. A total of 94% were still using their aids. The reasons
   given by those not wearing the aid were: batteries
   needed, repairs needed, no help to hearing, regained
   hearing, causes headaches, ear mold causes soreness,
   cumbersome, too noisy, causes nervous strain, and
   public disapproval of aid.

2. A change of hearing was suspected by 33%.

3. Difficulty in obtaining batteries, presumably through
   Veteran's Administration, was experienced by 24%.

4. Difficulty in obtaining satisfactory repair service
   had troubled 9%.

5. A total of 23% reported that they have been refused
   a job or have been unsuccessful in holding a job
   because of their hearing loss.

6. To the question, "How much has speechreading helped
   you to understand conversation?" 52% answered "greatly",
   35% "moderately" and 13% "slightly".

7. The study of speechreading has been continued since
   discharge by 45%; we assume this to be in the form
   of individual practice rather than formal instruction.

8. Suggestions for improving the program here included:
   (a) more speechreading, (b) more acquaintance with
   the workings of Veterans Administration, (c) more
   practice with the hearing aid, and (d) higher disability pension.

Lederer and Hardy argue strongly for a translation of the
military programs into civilian clinics and clinical programs. They write;

> By and large, there seems to be no apparent reason why
> the approach and the methodology developed in the ser-
> vice hearing centers cannot be applied to civilian
> hearing clinics. The translation needs only boldness
> and the resolution of interested professional groups.
>
> We believe that the naval principles and methods of
> aural rehabilitation described, based as they are on
> a wealth of practical experience in the field, provide
> an archetype for the clinical treatment and training
> of those with aural disability.
>
> The necessary steps in the procedure of examination,
> the evaluation and selection of hearing aids, the
> retraining of residual hearing with the use of an
> aid, and the development of skill in speechreading
> are clearcut. There are other ways of performing
> some of the tasks described here, but these have
> survived by reason of a successful demonstration,
> and this under conditions not always ideal.

Carhart talked on "An Integrated Program of Aural
Rehabilitation from the Military Point of View". These programs saw a joining of forces for the first time of several
specialists. There was little restriction from above; therefore, the programs were not GI (slang meaning Government
Issue). The centers had control of all aspects of the patients. The goal was to return the adults to civilian life
in a way fitted to carry on as normal an existence as possible. There was little or no pressure to return the men to
active duty.

The four centers (Deshon, Borden, Hoff, and the
Philadelphia Naval Hospital) combined to run a rehabilitation
program without any one group laying down rules for the
others. Each developed its own details. This allowed comparisons and a weighing of conclusions. The programs were
initiated in 1943. The Army program started at Walter Reed
but was moved to Deshon General Hospital in Butler,
Pennsylvania. There, the total personnel in the rehabilitation program was about 75. The patient admittance varied
from about 21 per month up to a peak of about 280. The load

of patients in the hospital varied from a couple hundred
to about 700. Since Deshon had 1700 beds, 700 was a sizeable
portion of the hospital.
        The program was housed in two buildings. One build-
ing had a large number of small rooms for lip reading, auditory training, et cetera, and two classrooms. The other
building had more offices for training, offices for the
administrative staff, plus testing rooms (six sound rooms,
etc.).

General Considerations

        The desire at all centers was to integrate the person
and eliminate the loss. The groups being handled were young
adults who had passed the entrance examinations. Practically,
this meant men who had enough language for everyday life and
a reasonable amount of hearing; therefore, there was no concern with the congenitally deaf nor the geriatric population.
A very few had several years in a school for the deaf.
        Carhart felt it was important to know the group in
order to understand the program. The group then were mature
men with their lives ahead of them. By and large, they had
moderate hearing losses. Army regulations and GI factors led
to the philosophy: If you take an average adult and concen-
trate, your efforts can do a lot in a hurry. The educators
who had been drafted or commissioned into the programs said
that it could not be done in a short time. However, it was
a short-term program; the average time at Deshon was ten
weeks, and for other programs it was "even less".
        One of the problems that Carhart saw with the mili-
tary programs was eccentricities of the commanding officers.
One called the men patients, which gave the staff personnel
little control, while another would treat them as GI's.
Carhart felt the retraining was more effective under the latter circumstances.

Aural Rehabilitation Program at Deshon

        The program at Deshon involved the following steps.
        Initial Phase. First, each person was processed
through admissions. Then he was given a thorough physical
and complete otological examination. This was followed by
an audiological assessment, which involved pure tone test by
air and bone conduction, and a speech threshold test with
records or by live voice. There was also an interview
series, which was sometimes done in depth with one person,

and in other instances a series of interviews. Most of the
men did not need ear treatment, but frequently they received
other minor treatments.

Program for giving insight into own difficulty. One
aspect of this part of the program included a series of lectures; e.g., medical lectures on anatomy and pathology of the
ear and on hearing and hearing loss, and lectures on hearing
aids, etc. The other aspect of this part of the program was
designed to get them to talk about their problem. There were
opportunities for the men to consult with staff members if
they wished to do so.

Orientation to hearing aids. About 9,000 aids were
issued during the war. It was necessary to break down the
antagonism toward hearing aids and establish what they could
do for the men. Typically, the men who came into the center
did not want hearing aids, but left wanting them. The interviews did a lot of good. They established formal and informal procedures to help the individual adjust to amplified
speech. At some of the rehabilitation centers, the hearing
aids were issued and put on quickly; others held orientation
programs first. At Deshon, the earmold was made early, but
the men used loaners from the Hearing Aid Library. Carhart
felt that, in one way or another, each individual must be
given extensive experience with amplified speech.

Selection of hearing aids. The purpose was to find
the most useful aid for each patient, and each patient's
needs differed. There were common features in the four
programs; namely, (a) there were a wide variety of brands
available as well as considerable variety within instruments
(8 to 12 instruments), and (b) there was adequate technical
staff and test techniques. There were also wide differences
in philosophies. At Borden, and also part of the time at
Hoff, the individual was fit quickly with a hearing aid and
then trained with his own instrument. In the opposite philosophy, the patient first adjusted to the facts of the aids,
and a training period preceded the actual issuance of the aid.
The "quick fitting" system used free field pure tone speech
tests with and without aids. The schedule at Borden called
for the aid-on-the-man in 72 hours. One of the problems at
all centers was maintaining a mass production procedure to
take care of the number of men involved and yet taking care
of each person as an individual.

At Deshon, they had an initial interview and took an
earmold impression. Ideally, each patient had an earmold in
48 to 72 hours. The fit of the earmold was checked carefully
and instructions were given on what was to happen next. At
this time a second pure tone and speech threshold test was

given. At the next session five to nine hearing aids were
selected for trial. Various aids were attached to the earmold and tried in an informal manner. A list of probably
useable aids was prepared, and the individual was taken directly to the Hearing Aid Library where he checked out the
first aid on the list. He kept this aid for 24 hours. He
was required to attend one listening hour and to prepare a
rating sheet on the aid (the listening hours ran every hour
of the day). He then returned his aid and drew another on
his list for 24 hours. This continued until he had worn each
of the aids on his list. Out of the aids he had tried, three
were selected and each aid was evaluated (one hour). (My
notes are not clear on whether one hour was spent with each
aid or one hour was devoted to the three.) Then the person
was told which aid suited him best, and later in the day that
aid was issued to him. If two aids were equal, the patient
was given his choice.

A total of 3,600 cases were seen at Deshon, and 2,600
of them were issued hearing aids.

Educational Program. The philosophy was to retrain
the person's communicative habits so he could best get along
in a hearing world; this was meant to minimize or eliminate
the hearing loss. It was generally recognized, among the
centers, that speaking and hearing are closely related.
Thus, they all focused on training of speaking, hearing, and
lip reading. Some places emphasized group work and others
focused on individual training.

The Lip Reading training varied among the four
centers. Although Carhart did not discuss it in his lectures
at the Symposium, the differences were to be expected. For
instance, Miriam Pauls (now Hardy) was in charge of Speech
Reading at the Philadelphia Naval Hospital, and she had been
trained in the Jena Method by Bunger, while Mrs. Nitchie,
wife of E. B. Nitchie, was on the staff at Deshon. In these
lectures Carhart did not discuss the lip reading program at
Deshon.

Carhart stated that auditory training was a challenge
because there were no established procedures for this type
of group (actually, compared to the literature on lip reading
and speech correction, he might have said that there was
little or nothing to give direction to any auditory training
program. At that time Goldstein had written The Acoustic
Method, Wright had made some suggestions, but, as he said,
what little there was had been directed at deaf children).
Each center developed its own training material, but all
goals were to make the patient as proficient as possible in
using his residual hearing. Each person was given tests

through group aids and without aids, not for the purpose of defining each individual's capacity but for defining what work needed to be done.

Whenever possible, at Deshon, the men were given auricular training to develop tolerance to loud sounds and to improve discrimination before they were issued aids. The staff felt that the listening hour was very important to the men in the program. The men became accustomed to amplified sound in everyday use and also in "The Hour". It gave the men full insight into what an aid would do for him and what problems he would have with tolerance of loud sounds and in discriminating speech. Through this each man learned the limitations of all aids and then would not blame his own aid. The listening hour was designed to focus his attention on various types of listening tasks and on gross discrimination. He rated each aid on 13 to 14 different things.

Once the aid was issued, each man was retested to see what his performance was with his own aid. He went on a training program which lasted from one to six weeks. He listened to music, to records, to newscasts, to radio programs, etc. Eventually he was given a discrimination proficiency examination on speech sounds. Some men were good enough that they did not get this program. Carhart was convinced that the training given in advance of the issuance of the aid was responsible for this success.

They learned that the men had difficulty bridging the gap between the quiet and unstressed listening situations in the centers and the listening requirements of everyday life. Eventually, they developed special types of training to help in this transition. They used ambient noises and made the men work and listen in noise. They also gave some localization training.

At Deshon, they used a sound treated room and installed six loud speakers, one on the ceiling, one on the floor, and one on each side wall. Sound could be put through one or more speakers in any combination. Carhart stated that there were four goals in the auditory training program at the Philadelphia Naval Hospital. These were: (a) to condition the patient to all types of auditory sounds, (b) to teach the patient to use the aid in everyday listening situations, (c) to help the person to understand his own loss, and (d) to acquaint him with the problems he might have with his hearing aid after he was out of service, such as how to get batteries from Veterans Administration, how to troubleshoot the aid, etc.

As with auditory training, there also was no precedence for planning the speech training. The original

assumption had been that speech would deteriorate with war
deafness and that recent loss cases needed an insurance program in which they developed a consciousness of good speech.
However, most of the men at the hospital had moderate hearing
losses, and with hearing aids, the deterioration did not
occur. Eventually, the speech training came to focus on
three types of handicaps. For the recent loss cases in which
the loss was moderate or moderately severe, the emphasis was
on adjusting to hearing their own speech and on sharpening
their speech habits. For individuals with severe to total
loss of hearing, emphasis was placed on monitoring their own
speech through kinesthetic clues plus whatever auditory clues
they could use. Speech was given high priority in this
group in order to prevent the development of bad speaking
habits. The third group was made up of indivudals who had
had hearing losses for many years and came to the center with
consequent defective speech. It appeared that these men
were speaking as they heard themselves. The speech problems
in this group was more than articulatory. Training focused
on avoiding slurring the endings of words. Usually there
was also need for voice improvement and training. Even with
a hearing aid these individuals were not able to monitor
their speech adequately. Apparently the hearing/speech problem had existed for too long to make quick corrections.

My notes on Carhart's series of two or three lectures
on the aural rehabilitation centers ends abruptly at this
point. I am surprised because his lectures were always carefully planned and timed. Yet my notes lack his typical
summary.

By way of summary, I think it is appropriate to state
that the staff members of the aural rehabilitation centers
were, by and large, satisfied with the retraining programs
and with the benefits provided to the hearing servicemen who
passed through the programs. It is unlikely that many, if
any, centers which try to offer aural rehabilitation today
are as satisfied with their efforts. In conclusion, I will
mention some of the differences in the World War II programs
and the programs of today.

Probably the greatest single difference is the fact
that the men were all full-time in service, that their job
was to participate in aural rehabilitation, and that learning to live with a hearing loss was their sole concern for
from four to eight weeks. This stands in sharp contrast to
programs today where the participants come in once a week for
one or two hours or, at most, come in two or three times a
week for an hour. The differences are obvious, and I will
not labor them. I wonder what success we might be having if,

from the beginning, aural rehabilitation was a requirement
to the acquisition of a hearing aid and if participation had
been set at a minimum of eight hours a day for four weeks?
We tend to think that participation would be impossible with
these requirements, but heart attacks, accidents, alcoholism,
drug withdrawal, etc., take individuals away from work for
four weeks or more, and it is accepted. It is unfortunate
that such a plan was never tried with the civilian
population.

One cannot have listened to these three men or have
read their reports without being impressed with the emphasis
they placed on treating the whole person. Perhaps the emphasis on mental hygiene, the focus on a person who wears a
hearing aid, not a person who is normal but cannot hear well,
and or group discussion of the problems of adjustment were
emphasized because there were psychologists and psychiatrists
on the staff, but all of us who have tried to serve the hearing impaired know that the fitting of a hearing aid is not
aural rehabilitation. In the clinic the hearing aid may be
judged by decibels of gain and percentage of discrimination
in quiet and in noise, but in life the test is more likely to
be the ability to hold the present work position or to be
judged qualified for promotion. I believe the emphasis on
total readjustment rather than hearing aid manipulation was
correct. However, it is easy to see that the objective hearing aid fitting procedure was easier to carry over into
hearing clinics than were the listening hour, the group
speechreading, and the sharing of experiences.

Grouping the hearing impaired on the basis of common
degrees of hearing losses, common educational and intellectual levels, and other common interests was standard practice
in most of the centers. Lederer spoke of eight clinics per
million population to serve the twenty thousand hearing
impaired. He felt a prime form of these clinics would be the
University Medical Clinic. This organization would treat and
retrain persons handicapped by defective speech and hearing,
would educate professional personnel and disseminate public
information, and would carry out research on every aspect of
speech and hearing including reeducation. He thought that
"Aural rehabilitation offers an excellent opportunity for a
much needed and progressive type of philanthropy". There
are a number of innovative ways in which the Clinics in a
metropolitan area could alternate or share programs offering
group aural rehabilitation.

As one attempts to assess whether the principles and
procedures of the World War II Centers represent a situation
unique to wartime or have application to civilian clinics,

the apparent commonality of a sudden and recent hearing loss
would appear to be unique to wartime. However, both Canfield
and Lederer point out that large numbers of men who were
routed to the centers had had hearing losses when they
entered service. Apparently, sizeable numbers of both army
and navy personnel had otosclerosis. Nowhere does one find
a statement that the rehabilitation program could have been
eliminated for the personnel who had long standing hearing
losses. On the contrary, intensive aural rehabilitation is
likely to be more important for the individual who has become habituated to devious forms of dealing with the hearing
loss. Certainly the program would be different for the
sudden loss cases from the program for the persons who suddenly decide something must be done, but I do not believe
that these facts obviate the good principles of the military
programs.

I find the emphasis on the production of speech--
including voice, articulation, and phonetics--and the emphasis on speechreading to be thought provoking. Carhart
admitted that the training in speech production was introduced to prevent deterioration in speech which did not occur.
However, the training continued, and one gets the impression
that the focus on the production of speech was incidentally
beneficial to the aided reception of speech and to acquiring
speechreading skills. I do not rule out the possibility that
it remained in the program simply because the original plan-
ners thought it ought to be there. Undoubtedly, it was
simpler to continue the program rather than to drop it, find
something else to use to fill the time, and to reassign or
discharge the personnel. Certainly, I do not know of any
research then or since which relates to speech training as a
routine part of aural rehabilitation.

Obviously, both the staff personnel and the hearing-
impaired servicemen thought that training in speechreading
was extremely valuable. In the questionnaire referred to by
Lederer and Hardy, additional training in speechreading was
one of the suggestions made by the individuals who had been
through the program. The emphasis on speechreading, by both
groups, is a little hard to understand from our present point
of view when much less emphasis is being placed on it. Perhaps we should reconsider our programs of aural rehabilitation and give blocks of training to speech, speechreading,
speech discrimination and listening projects, at least until
we have evidence that another way would produce better
results.

There are many aspects of the World War II programs
that seem to warrant reconsideration. However, I find it

especially interesting that none of the three men reviewed
here made any mention of speech discrimination of the PB-50
type, according to my notes or in the Lederer and Hardy
article. The speech reception test was mentioned as the best
measure of the loss in hearing and of the benefit derived
from the hearing aid. It is true that the PB-50 lists were
not available when the programs started, but they became
available during the life of the programs and they were used
at Deshon at least. The change in emphasis from then to now
may or may not mean that we are off on the wrong track, but,
at least, it appears that the early programs were successful
without the use of and the emphasis on speech discrimination
as it is presently measured.

When considering the material I have presented, I
wondered if it were appropriate for a Symposium on Aural
Rehabilitation for the Elderly. I think it is. If we assume
that the average age of the men in service, when these aural
rehabilitation programs started in 1943, was about 25, then
35 years later the average age of the servicemen of World War
II is approaching 60 and they are now about to become the
elderly. Perhaps we can use what was learned from a few of
the hearing impaired from their generation to help the
larger number, of their generation, who now have or shortly
will develop hearing impairments.

Chapter 2

Aural Rehabilitation for the
Elderly: State of the Art

MIRIAM A. HENOCH, PH. D.

When I first decided to take on the task of preparing a presentation on the state of the art in aural rehabilitation of the elderly, I envisioned a relatively simple task;
one which would involve a few hours of perusing through the
relevant research and methodologies dealing with the topic.
With this in mind, and with symposium arrangements, not to
mention the usual activities of a university professor needing constant attention, the writing task was procrastinated.
Then one day I glanced at my calendar and went into that
panic state that procrastinators like myself often experience. The symposium was only a few weeks away and I had yet
to walk the short distance to our university library to begin
my perusing. I did not worry too much however, I knew a few
late nights in the library would see the job completed.
My first night in the library began with the *Deafness,
Speech and Hearing Abstracts* dating back to 1960 stacked
neatly in front of me. The first two volumes produced little
results. However, I was not too concerned--I had eighteen
more volumes to go. But when volume number five had been set
aside and I had found a grand total of four articles relating
to the topic, I felt more than a little concerned. My concern turned to alarm after the tenth volume and then pure and
simple dismay when I had finished with the 1978 editions.
All of these emotions were not directed to the lack of references to include in my presentation, they were directed to
the lack of attention that has been focused on the communication problems of the elderly as a result of hearing
impairment.
Now keep in mind that I am not discussing aural rehabilitation in general. The information available on the
habilitation and rehabilitation of children with hearing loss
is overwhelming; and lipreading lessons for adults have been
available since the turn of the century. I am talking specifically about rehabilitation for elderly adults, individuals

who are 65 years of age and older and whose hearing loss is
most probably a result of presbycusis.

Ever since I was a student in audiology I have known
that aural rehabilitation as it relates to the elderly person
has not been a major area of concentration for the majority
of speech and hearing professionals. However, it was not
brought to mind with such impact until I began to look at
what has actually been done. Another interesting finding, at
least for me, was that up until the last two or three years,
a great deal of the information available has been published
in journals that are not widely read by speech and hearing
professionals. One of the journals which has published a
number of articles is *Geriatrics*, a journal primarily directed to the gerontologist. Now I feel it is extremely important that professionals outside of the speech and hearing
field be made aware of the hearing problems of the elderly
and how to deal with them. I also know that audiologists
and speech/language pathologists have little time to read the
multitude of journals in their own field, much less the journals of other fields, no matter how closely they may be
related. Since a number of the articles in *Geriatrics* dealt
with the communication problems of the elderly in nursing
homes, I began to see why so many of us in my profession have
been lacking in our knowledge of the problems specific to
this particular population. The information has been there,
but many of us have simply not been aware of its existence.

I believe the void of information in some of our own
professional journals may be the direct result of just where
we, the audiologists, have been in the past in our attention
to the rehabilitation needs of our senior citizens. Needless
to say that trend is changing. Audiologists, as well as
speech/language pathologists, are becoming more mindful of
the importance of improving all aspects of communication
function for the elderly. The Academy of Rehabilitative
Audiology devoted its summer meeting in 1976 to the geriatric
client. The trend in the last three or four years has been
to place more emphasis on the role of the audiologist as a
rehabilitationist rather than "a person who tests hearing".
However, it would still appear that our major focus in educational programs is on the rehabilitation of children rather
than elderly adults.

The American Speech and Hearing Association requires
that students concentrating in the area of audiology receive
a minimum of 50 clock hours of supervised practicum in aural
rehabilitation. In a typical one year masters degree program, 50 hours is <u>all</u> they get and probably 95% of those
hours are spent working with children; hardly enough to give

one the proficiency he or she needs to develop the special
knowledge and confidence necessary for working effectively
with an elderly population. It is no wonder then that the
majority of students who are graduating from our universities are directing their time and talents to other, more
secure endeavors.

I noted with interest a statement in Dr. Alpiner's
new book, Handbook of Adult Rehabilitative Audiology (1978),
that all of the hearing rehabilitation programs reported for
senior citizens are under the auspices of university speech
and hearing departments. To quote him directly, "If the need
to expose students to geriatric audiology did not exist, it
is doubtful that there would be many meaningful programs for
our older citizens in the United States". I honestly do not
know how many training programs have geriatric audiology on
an equal par with other aspects of their audiology program,
the fact that the programs for aural rehabilitation exist
only in university settings leads me to believe that it is
too few. If more programs did incorporate geriatric audiology into their curriculum, then perhaps more of our graduating students would be incorporating it into their own professional settings, be it community speech and hearing
center, private practice, indeed, even making audiology for
the elderly an area of specialization.

So what is the state of the art at this point in
time? Where are we in terms of training the elderly to participate in the joy of communication with others in spite of
the hearing problem that is a common occurrence in the aging
process? Even though we are far from where we should be, we
have made a start, be it ever so humble.

In my own mind, I think of aural rehabilitation of
the elderly as beginning with John Gaeth and "phonemic regression". I remember being intrigued with the term and its
definition as a graduate student here at North Texas State
University and even more so as a doctoral student under this
wise and excellent teacher at Wayne State University. I say
it begins there for me because the fact that problems other
than peripheral degeneration of the auditory mechanism can
and do play a part in the hearing problems of the elderly.
This has certainly made me aware that the procedures and
methods we use in our therapy techniques for this population
must be different than those we incorporate into our programs
for younger age groups.

Yet in a number of programs that have been described,
the only major modifications of the traditional aural rehabilitation procedures are to take the program to the clients,
and to make "significant others", e.g., family members,

nursing home personnel, etc., more aware and informed of
hearing loss and how to deal with it. One such traditional
approach is speechreading. Hardick, et al. (1970), told us
that there was a significant relationship between visual
acuity and lipreading performance. Yet a majority of the
programs that have been described rely mainly on lipreading
drills for their elderly clients. We know vision is another
sensory modality that grows considerably poorer with age.
Trying to read lips one cannot see clearly must be a most
discouraging endeavor.

   This does not necessarily mean that the visual channel is completely lost to the elderly hearing impaired
person. It means we must change the traditional lipreading
approaches to something that can be used in a more meaningful way. Dean Garstecki is doing some very interesting
research on situational cues in visual speech perception
which may indeed facilitate the rehabilitation process of
the geriatric client. What I find particularly appealing is
the use of the term *Visual Speech Perception* as opposed to
lipreading or speechreading, because the former term takes
into account the total of the visual communication process,
not merely one aspect of it.

   Hull (1977), pointed out that although elderly persons can learn as easily as young persons, they have some
problems in the speed of processing linguistic information.
The speed of auditory processing, synthesis, and sequential
storage are all retarded by the central auditory components
of presbycusis. In spite of this knowledge very little
attention has been focused on how to deal with these problems
in the rehabilitative process. I believe that Bob
McCroskey's research focusing on temporal auditory behavior
in elderly individuals might lead us into new directions for
our rehabilitative procedures.

   One of the most encouraging aspects of the aural
rehabilitative audiology programs being developed by a number
of university hearing and speech clinics, is the recognition
that in order to serve this population most effectively, the
programs must be taken to them. It is often difficult, if
not impossible, to get elderly people interested in coming to
a speech and hearing clinic for aural rehabilitation. Even
those who are still able to transport themselves with relative ease cannot be motivated to spend an hour or two a week
in a hearing and speech clinic. As I expect Jerry Alpiner
will point out, psychological factors have a great deal to do
with this. Many elderly individuals live in nursing homes,

therefore the means to travel to a speech and hearing clinic is very often denied to these individuals. This problem has been dealt with quite effectively in a number of programs in which the audiologist travels to the nursing home or senior citizen center and conducts the program on-site. In the majority of such programs, the first phase is a hearing screening. I have found in my own experiences that this initial screening helps accomplish three important functions; 1) identifies a hearing loss that may be handicapping to communication, 2) gives the audiologist a chance to be viewed as someone who really cares about the problem which in turn 3) serves as a motivational force for the hearing impaired elderly person.

The last two functions were accomplished by simply listening to the individuals talk about their hearing problem. I am beginning to believe that there is an inverse relationship between aging and listening. The older we get, the more tuned out those around us seem to become.

If an individual fails the hearing screening, the second phase of an aural rehabilitation program is most often a complete audiological evaluation. A hearing aid evaluation and fitting may be included in this phase if deemed appropriate. The third phase is generally spent with hearing aid orientation, lipreading and auditory training. The final phase generally deals with the counseling of family members as well as inservice training programs for nursing home staff or senior citizen staff personnel.

As ideal as this type of program is, in most cases it is not affordable to either client or audiologist. To my knowledge, no agency, federal or private pays for aural rehabilitation services. The majority of senior citizens cannot afford to pay for these services themselves. In some university clinics where these types of services might be provided free of charge, the problem of providing qualified staff to personally conduct such services or to supervise students to conduct such services is one which often appears to be unsolvable.

This does not mean that we cannot make such programs available to the people who need and want them, it simply means we have to search out all possible means of support and present a convincing case for the necessity of our services when we have located possible funding sources. In the past four or five years, professions other than speech and hearing have been focusing attention on the communication problems of the elderly. The administrative staffs of nursing homes and

personnel involved in senior citizen centers are realizing
the need for programs which identify handicapping hearing
loss and provide rehabilitative services. This is due in
part to the number of articles appearing in the journals
relative to gerontology. Also, the development of the
National Institute on Aging has provided a means by which
individuals can apply for funding to support various research
projects exploring many facets of the aging process, including communication problems.

While serving as an administrator for a hearing and
speech center in Detroit, Michigan, part of my responsibility
was to set up satellite programs for aural rehabilitation in
nursing homes and senior citizen centers. The biggest challenge was not in convincing these facilities of the need for
such services, but rather finding ways to support the staff
conducting the programs. I found several funding sources
which included, small grants from local philantropic organizations, grants from area agencies on aging, direct payment
from family members of the hearing impaired person, and in
some cases, nursing homes paid for the services out of their
operational budgets, particularly if the nursing home was
sponsored by a religious organization. Graduate students in
audiology from Wayne State University were often used in the
initial screening process. This enabled us to provide the
initial hearing screening phase of the program free of charge
to the nursing home or senior center.

Although we were able to provide screening services,
follow-up audiological services and aural rehabilitation out
of the money provided by our funding sources, we still lacked
the ability to provide hearing aids to those who needed them
if they were not eligible for Medicaid coverage. To solve
this problem we accumulated used hearing aids which were donated by the hearing and speech center clients as well as
hearing aid dealers. We had the hearing aids reconditioned
at a minimal cost, usually no more than $20.00. This expense
was borne by the person receiving the aid when possible.
When it was not possible, the aid was given on a permanent
loan basis, being returned to us only if the individual
could no longer use it.

My own experience has shown me that services can be
taken to elderly individuals in their own environment.
Services provided in this manner are usually more effective
and successful than those in which we attempt to convince the
elderly clients to come to us. Certainly available statistics point to the need for rehabilitative audiology for the
elderly.

The number of people who are now living to and beyond the age of 65 as compared to previous years is truly remarkable. For example, in 1900 about 4% of the total population in the United States was 65 years of age or older. That accounted for about three million people. Today approximately 10.9% of the total population falls in that age group. This amounts to about 23 million people. The U.S. Census Bureau predicts that by the year 2030 about 50 million people will be 65 years of age or older (DHEW, 1978). The number of people living beyond the age of 65 years of age has not been proportional to the total population growth, but has been greater. People are simply living longer and with continuing medical advances are capable of living productive, useful lives well beyond age 65.

Statistics compiled from the Metropolitan Life Insurance Company (1959) indicate that 129 persons per 1000 ranging in age from 65-74 suffer some degree of hearing impairment; the incidence in the 75 and over age group is 256 per 1000. That means out of the approximately 23 million persons who are now 65 years and over, about 8.8 million suffer some degree of hearing impairment.

About five million persons reside in nursing homes. It is estimated that as many as 90% of these individuals have a hearing loss which may interfere with communication (Hull, 1977). What affect can this degree of hearing loss have on the elderly person? Hull (1977) stated it quite dramatically: "Its impact upon communicative function of the aging person is often times overwhelming. The inability to hear and understand what others are saying can be the final blow toward the finality of aging. The frustration, embarrassment and resulting self-imposed isolation can, in the final analysis, lead to social and physical death."

What can we do to improve the state of the art? We can continue to do what the symposium participants have done and are continuing to do; be concerned and aware that the hearing problems of the elderly are not confined to the term "presbycusis" as defined in a basic audiology course. We can seek funding for research projects to develop more effective methods of rehabilitation. We who are educators in the field of audiology can make geriatric audiology as important to the overall training program as pediatric audiology, with equal practicum requirements.

I have found that working with the elderly is as much of a rewarding and as rich an experience as working with the very young child. The needs of each are quite different, but the ultimate goal remains the same: to provide an effective means of verbal expression and communication.

REFERENCES

1. Alpiner, J. G., Rehabilitation of the geriatric client. In J. G. Alpiner (Ed.), Handbook of Adult Rehabilitative Audiology. Baltimore: The Williams Wilkins Co., 1978.

2. Hardick, E. J., Oyer, H. J., & Irion, P. E., Lipreading performance as related to measurement of vision. *Journal of Speech and Hearing Research, 13,* 92-100, 1970.

3. Hull, R. H., Aural rehabilitation for the aging hearing impaired person, *Journal of the Academy of Rehabilitative Audiology, 10,* 46-50, 1977.

4. Metropolitan Life Insurance Company, *Statistical Bulletin, 40,* 1, 1959.

5. U.S. Department of Health, Education, and Welfare, Changes...research on aging and the aged. DHEW Publication No. (NIH) 78-85, 5-9, 1978.

Chapter 3

Aural Rehabilitation:
Philosophy, Rationale and Technique

JOHN C. COOPER, PH. D.

PHILOSOPHY

It would be impossible, within these time limitations, to cover all aspects of a philosophy, rationale, and
technique for aural rehabilitation of the elderly. What I do
hope to do is set the stage for the fine papers which follow
by providing a broad overview of the process. I start with
the philosophy because the assumptions that we make about
life govern all aspects of our behavior. I do not mean to
become involved in any esoteric issues. I believe that two
philosophical issues are relevant to aural rehabilitation.
They are 1) the issue of free-will versus the determinism and
2) the issue of the function of audiologists in a rehabilitation process.
The issue of free-will versus determinism has two
important dimensions. While somewhat afield of our discussion today, the first dimension is most obvious in the bumper
sticker "deaf babies can talk". This seems to imply that
will power, courage, and hard work will lead any hearing impaired child down the pathway to essentially normal aural
communication. It stands in dramatic contrast to those among
us who take the position that if there is no measurable hearing in the speech range it is unlikely that the deaf baby
will ever talk. In the first case, the optimism is based on
ignorance of, for example, radiographic studies which show
that a number of deaf babies simply do not have cochleas plus
a generalization to all deaf based on the few severely hearing impaired children who do operate with near normal aural
communication. In the second case, the pessimist may resign
a child to a purely manual method of communication in ignorance of, for example, Chuck Berlin's study (1978) which shows
that hearing above 8000 Hz may be the factor which allows for
the dramatic successes upon which the bumper sticker relies.
What appears to be an arguable point boils down to incomplete
knowledge on the part of both the optimist and the pessimist.

Closer to home we find individuals who still assert that
those with sensorineural hearing losses do poorly with hearing aids and, categorically, should not be given a hearing
aid evaluation. The important fundamental point is that I
believe behavior is governed and limited by specifiable factors even though we may not have complete knowledge of them.
Behavior results from determining factors not an act of will.
     The second dimension of the issue is the problem of
behavioral alternatives to a given set of stimulus inputs.
An assumption among those of us who might be classified as
determinists seems to be that only few responses are available under a given set of stimulus conditions. Even though
responses can be limited in the laboratory, this is not the
case in an ongoing day-to-day world. What masks as free will
is our failure to account for all influences and all behavioral alternatives. A variety of past experiences which may
be summarized in terms of net punishment or reward influences
a person's willingness to communicate. By understanding the
forces operating on an individual, we can manipulate stimuli
to permit the hearing impaired to come close to some theoretical optimum. However, they will choose among several behavioral alternatives and it is important to realize that one of
them is, in multiple choice format, "none of the above". In
part, their choice may be influenced by the posture taken by
the audiologist.
     Which brings me to the second philosophical issue
that I have chosen to discuss. Because of my own experiences
I caricaturize the audiologist's attitude about the hearing
impaired as being at one of two extremes. These are the God-
like giver of instructions or the knowledgeable and resource-
ful consultant.
     The important difference between the two has to do
with the status assigned to the patient. In the first case
the patient merely becomes an extension of the therapist's
realm of control.
     The therapist becomes a drill instructor and the pa-
tient one of several boots assigned to his care. Everything
goes well so long as the drill instructor can control the
environment. His task is simple: give a set of instructions
which the boots will memorize. The simpler the environment
can be kept, the fewer instructions need to be given and the
more smoothly the boots' life will go. Innovation, either in
environment or on the part of the boots, will do nothing more
than disrupt the smooth functioning of the platoon. It is a
truly excellent model if you are able to control the environ-

ment. At the opposite extreme the patient completely domi-
nates the picture. He becomes an individual faced with an
exceedingly complex environment which extends far beyond simple acoustic considerations. There are a variety of methods
by which he can bring some sort of order to his chaotic environment. He may do so on the basis of trial and error or he
may choose to enlist the services of some individual who has
faced these problems before and who may be able to short cut
his trial and error process. Let us presume that he chooses
to select a consultant, in this case one of us. He can reasonably expect that we have some knowledge of the problems
that he faces and that we have some reasonable, viable solutions for those problems. He cannot expect us to know the
details or ramifications of any of his specific problems,
only to understand the relevant underlying parameters which
govern the situation. He can expect us to provide him with
the principles and tools which will allow him to solve any
problem that he might face. He can also expect us to give
him some supervised practical experience in problem solving
to insure that he has acquired the proper information and the
technical skill to apply that information. I think you have
a broad idea of what I'm trying to get at. In one case, the
rehabilitationist presumes to save his patient. In the other
case the rehabilitationist is nothing more than a consultant
who is expected to provide the assistance necessary so that
the patient can save himself.

       How then to summarize my philosophy about aural re-
habilitation? I believe that all behavior, including communication, is related to present stimulus conditions as well as
past experience. I believe that an individual has more than
one alternative when faced with a reduced auditory environment and that he may need our specialized knowledge to assist
him in selecting the alternative which is best suited for his
current needs. I believe that the most long lasting method
for meeting a particular patient's needs is to insure that he
has the information and the opportunity to develop the skills
necessary to meet those needs. I believe it is our role to
provide the hearing impaired with that background. I remain
categorically opposed to the premise that rehabilitation must
be forced on anyone. I believe that there are some individuals who either cannot develop the resources necessary to
sustain their rehabilitation or who choose not to employ
their communication ability to a maximum. In the first case
we must accept failure and in the second we must accept their
choice.

RATIONALE

    A rationale for rehabilitation must presume that the
patient is interested in more efficient communication. This
may not be the case in the elderly but I will postpone a
discussion of what to do about lack of motivation until we
get to technique. Under any circumstances, there are three
groups of information which form the basis of the rationale:
an understanding of normal hearing, of abnormal hearing and
of rehabilitation alternatives.
    There are two aspects of normal hearing which bear
upon rehabilitation. The first is its physiology. The second is the psychoacoustics of normal hearing. Normal physiology involves four distinct steps between the acoustic signal in the environment and our subjective experience that
someone said such and such a word. Air pressure variations
are significantly modified and amplified by the conductive
mechanism which can be conceived of as extending from the
baffle effects of the head through to pressure variations
introduced into the cochlear fluid by the footplate of the
stapes. The complicated wave form of the acoustic signal is
analyzed in the cochlea so that we may roughly approximate
sound by conceiving of it as a series of spectral representa-
tions extending in time. This changing spectral representation is transmitted via the auditoric pathways to the cortex
where it is decoded, compared to some internal standard and
finally "recognized".
    The psychoacoustics of communication can also be
summarized in a relatively simple way. The basic information can be represented by the articulation function or performance intensity function which related performance in
some auditory discrimination task to the level of sound.
While the performance intensity function is familiar to all
of you, I will take the liberty of pointing out that the
shape of the function is clearly dependent upon the materials involved and the context in which they are presented.
As well, it is related to the amount of visual input and/or
competing noise which may partly obscure the signal. Figure
1 points out these two qualifications.

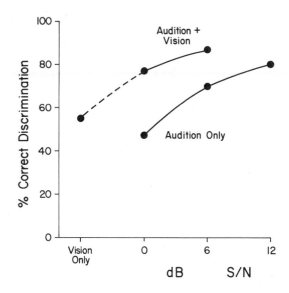

FIG. 1. *Performance intensity functions for auditory and audiovisual presentations from normal hearers.*

The material involved in collecting this data was the Modified Rhyme Test (Cooper & Langley, 1978), recorded on video tape, and played back through an audiometer with or without the opportunity to see a television monitor. The subjects were normal hearing individuals naive to any kind of auditory testing or to any formal understanding of the factors involved in communication. Purely auditory performance improved with increasing signal to noise ratio. As expected, the addition of visual input improved scores at any given signal to noise ratio. The data point on the far left was the subjects' performance without any auditory input. It is clear that even naive listeners use vision to supplement their audition under difficult listening conditions. In fact, it would appear that the addition of vision is roughly equivalent to a 12 dB increase in the signal to noise ratio.

Hearing loss in the elderly is likely to alter normal physiology in two major ways. At a cochlear level, frequency

analysis of the acoustic signal is distorted by alternations
in sensitivity and, therefore, alternations in the spectrum
of the signal available for transmission to the cortex. As
well, one may find that intensity input-output relationships
are altered such that sounds which are reasonably tolerable
to the normal auditory system may become intolerable. Secondly, the transmission system is altered. The alterations
introduce distortions such that we find a reduction in the
total information transmitting capability exhibited in such
phonomena as phenomenic regression and performance intensity
rollover (Gaeth, 1948; Gang, 1976). On the basis of presbycusis alone, there are no consistent alternations in the
processing of pressure variations as they travel from the
environment through to the footplate of the stapes. Decoding
and interpretation functions in the cortex may be effected
although these disabilities are generally not categorized as
being auditory in nature.
     Psychoacoustic manifestations of these changes in
physiology are best demonstrated graphically. Figure 2 is a
rough abstraction of the performance intensity function of a
normal individual on the left and that from a hypothetical
patient on the right.

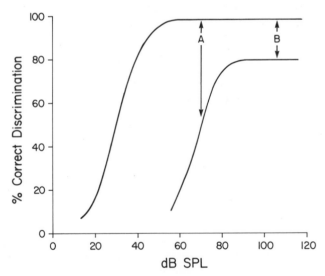

FIG. 2. Performance intensity functions for
normal (A) and hypothetical hearing impaired
indicating performance differences at conversational (A) and maximum (B) levels.

The difference denoted by the letter A indicates the reduced communication efficiency at normal conversational level which results from reduced auditory sensitivity. More importantly, the performance intensity function reaches a plateau which is significantly below the 100% which would be expected in normal hearing individuals. This reduced plateau level may reflect the reduced transmission capacity of the auditory pathways and/or altered frequency response in the cochlea which prevents critical speech information from being transmitted to the cortex. A more dramatic alteration which can occur in the performance intensity function is shown in Figure 3.

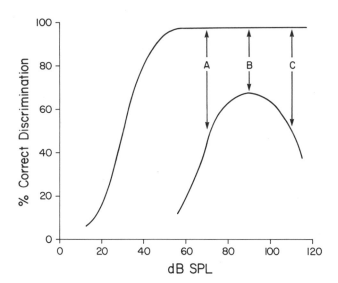

FIG. 3. Performance intensity functions for normal (A) and hypothetical hearing impaired indicating performance differences at conversational (A), maximum (B) and rollover (C) levels.

Once again dimension B shows a reduced capability at the high point of the function. The most important feature is the rollover indicated by dimension C where, at high levels of presentation, the patient's discrimination is reduced back to his performance at normal conversational level. This rollover is most probably associated with deteriorating

auditory pathways from the cochlea to the cortex. Figure 4
demonstrates possible alterations which may occur in the
subjective responses to intensity.

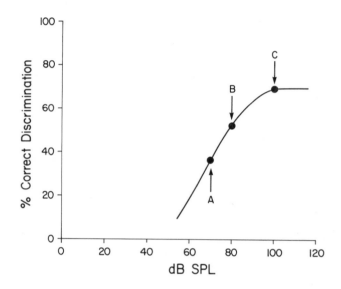

FIG. 4. *Performance intensity function for*
hypothetical hearing impaired indicating
conversational (A), comfort (B) and discom-
fort (C) levels.

Point A indicates normal conversational level. Point B indicates a level which the patient considers comfortable.
Notice that it is well below the plateau of the performance
intensity function. Point C indicates a level of discomfort.
Notice that this level of discomfort occurs at the beginning
of his area of maximum performance. You can imagine the difficulties that might be encountered in managing this hypothetical patient. He is capable of a doubling of his discrimination ability from approximately 35 to 70%. However, to
achieve the improvement he must subject himself to sounds
which are intolerably loud.

     Two other aspects of the changes in psychoacoustic
function can be demonstrated by way of an audiometric representation. Figure 5 presents an abstraction of the range of
speech sounds as might be displayed on an audiogram.

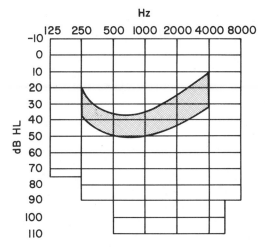

FIG. 5. Audiometric representation of the range of speech sounds.

Figure 6 presents the mean audiogram for males between 65 and 75 years of age superimposed upon the representation of speech sounds. Notice that approximately 1/4 of the speech area is not heard as a result of the altered sensitivity of the cochlea.

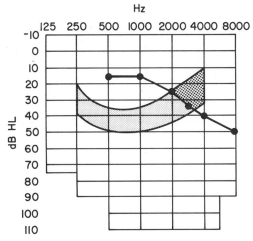

FIG. 6. Audiometric representation of the range of speech sounds with the average audiogram of 65 to 75 year old males superimposed. Cross hatched area indicates inaudible stimuli.

Figure 7 points up the compound effect of reduced hearing
and noise upon the information available to a hearing impaired person.

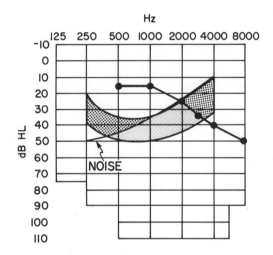

FIG. 7. *Audiometric representation of the
range of speech sounds with the average
audiogram of 65 to 75 year old males and
typical background noise superimposed.
Cross hatched area indicates inaudible
stimuli.*

As we have seen, noise can interfere with a normal individual's discrimination. Under these conditions of noise a
normal hearing individual would hear some 70% of the available speech sounds, the remainder being masked by the noise.
The masked portion of the speech involves relatively uni-
formative sounds and does not interfere with the important
consonant sounds. However, when the noise is combined with
a hearing loss, an individual is left with less than 1/2
of the original signal. Therefore, based on no more than
this simplistic analysis, we can predict that a hearing impaired person will encounter significantly more difficulty
in noise than normal hearers.
        The consequences of this review of normal and abnor-
mal hearing should be obvious for rehabilitation. Ignoring
the issue of a person's desire to communicate and focusing
solely on the alteration of psychoacoustic function which

results from hearing loss, rehabilitation alternatives boil
down to amplification, supplementing auditory cues via lipreading, and instituting environmental controls, primarily
noise reduction in the communication environment.

TECHNIQUE

From what has been said so far rehabilitation may
seem deceptively easy. Unfortunately, it can be a tedious
and often seemingly impossible task. To begin with, we need
to establish some criteria for determining whether or not
rehabilitation is necessary or possible. We need not go
through the details of an audiological evaluation here. However, several features of a rehabilitative evaluation should
be mentioned. First of all, some estimate of the current
level of communication needs to be established. Ideally,
the estimate should include three facets. Initially, measures of understanding conversationally loud speech should
be obtained in both quiet and noise with both an auditory
and audiovisual signal. Secondly, the individuals potential
for communication should be established by obtaining performance intensity functions in quiet and noise, with and without visual input. Fortunately, for those of us with a tight
schedule, a complete matrix of results is not always possible or necessary. Lastly, a clear picture should be had of
the particular communication difficulties that the patient
is experiencing. This should include the frequency of encountering difficulty, the environments involved, the individuals with whom communication is found to be difficult,
and the importance of these difficult situations to the patient's overall pattern of living.

If any of the conversationally loud auditory presentations produce poorer than normal performance, rehabilitation is indicated. If any of the performance intensity
functions demonstrate an improvement in communication efficiency with amplification, then a hearing aid is likely to
be a part of the overall rehabilitation technique. In laying the ground work for hearing aid acceptance by the patient it is crucial that he understand that hearing aids do
not restore normal hearing. At best, the patient can only
hope that amplification will provide a significant reduction
in his communication difficulties. The failure to distinguish between an improvement and a return to normal hearing
lies at the root of many expressions of hearing aid dissat-
isfaction. Assuming the patient is willing to deal with
improvement rather than perfection, the audiologist faces a
rather confusing morass of suggestions for selecting

appropriate amplification. At one extreme you find the advocates of high fidelity for everyone. At the other extreme
are those promoting a mirror-the-audiogram technique. I
find no convincing evidence for either of the two extreme
positions but readily acknowledge that getting commercially
available amplification which meets either's specification
is practically impossible. Let us look at some of the limitations of the two positions. The hi-fi-for-all advocates
meet their nemesis in the steeply falling audiogram which
may require an amplifying system to deliver 90 dB in the
3000 Hz range to insure audibility of those components of
speech while in doing so speech components in the 250 Hz
range would be over amplified. Given the variability of comfort levels across the frequency range, the mirror-the-audiogram folks may also run into the same problem of exceeding
comfort levels if they try to restore normal sensitivity at
all frequencies. Even if levels of discomfort were not an
issue, they would run into considerable difficulty in finding a practical method by which to tailor amplification.
This is so because of the variable and often unpredictable
effects associated with physically mounting a hearing aid on
a human being. As a sampler, consider the following list:
the head baffle effect, the effect of microphone location,
the effect of the ear mold and the degree to which it is
vented, the effect of tubing including both its length and
diameter, the relative inflexibility of manipulating the
frequency response of the hearing aid's electronics, the model to model variability within a particular hearing aid man-
ufacturing run, and last, but certainly not least, the
failure of standard electroacoustic measuring techniques to
match the typical coupling of an ear mold to an ear drum.
If you are beginning to feel uneasy about our ability to tailor the response of a hearing aid, then you have gotten the
point. Nonetheless, most of us feel that we can make some
reasonable approximation of fitting a hearing aid to a hearing impaired person. That approximation appears to be some
compromise between the two extremes. We amplify enough to
insure that the overall, as-worn frequency response brings
speech into the range of audibility without causing the patient undue discomfort.

 I would like to state a cautionary note for anyone
who is intimately involved in fitting hearing aids. It has
to do with the fact that hearing aids appear to be malfunctioning about half of the time. To deal with hearing aids
and be unable to specify their electroacoustic performance
is sheer madness. Hearing aid specifications may be of
little, if any, value in actually fitting a hearing aid.

They are, however, essential to determining the function of a particular hearing aid. Since hearing aids and automobiles and washing machines do malfunction, it is imperative that a hearing aid's performance be compared to its specifications in the event of any complaint so that the hearing aid's problems can be separated from the patient's.

Aside from the many technical problems associated with the selection of a hearing aid's frequency response, other decisions have to be made. The physical configuration of the hearing aid must meet a particular patient's needs. In the case of the elderly, for example, a body hearing aid may be required not because of its greater potential for amplification but simply because of the larger controls which it typically possesses. Reduced manual dexterity or visual acuity may make the typical ear level aid physically unmanageable. To CROS or not to CROS is closely associated with a third practical consideration, the selection of ear mold configuration to provide a maximum of comfort with a minimum of feedback.

Lastly, and most importantly for the patient, a hearing aid must be accompanied with instruction in its use and maintenance. The patient must be able to troubleshoot his aid including battery checks, cord and receiver checks when appropriate, and ear mold and tubing checks. He should have an idea of what are normal and abnormal levels of internal noise, including noise which may be contributed by the progressive deterioration of a volume control. Instruction in hearing aid use should include setting the volume control. If the person has a comfort level which is below the maximum of his performance intensity function, it should include instructions to attempt progressively higher settings of the volume control. After fitting and testing of the hearing aid while worn by the patient, the volume control should be marked to indicate both minimal and maximal settings necessary for efficient communication.

If the evaluative steps demonstrate below normal audiovisual performance, and probably under any circumstances, lipreading instruction should be considered. I must emphasize that my view of such instruction does not extend to an interminable series of psycho-therapeutic meetings. While there are good reasons to have ongoing "lipreading" classes, basic patient instruction is not one of them. I mean some ten sessions or so. That instruction should begin with a broad overview of the capabilities and limitations of lipreading. Instruction continues with defining what can be seen, what cannot be seen and how the visable aspects of speech can be confused. These periods of didactic

presentations are interspursed with periods of practice both
in the classroom and in home assignments such as watching
news broadcasts with minimal audio levels or with the volume
set at zero. Practice sessions in the classroom should be
graded, becoming progressively more comprehensive and difficult. Because of the ambiguities associated with lipreading
cues and to facilitate adjustment to and use of amplification, practice should certainly include audiovisual presentations. If these are too easy for class members then noise
should be included as part of the acoustic environment.

While on the topic of listening in noise, it is well
to mention that there is no conclusive evidence that listening in noise will improve communication efficiency. Two
studies bear on the point. The first involved the auditory
discrimination of recorded control tower traffic (Unpublished
Data, Brooks AFB). The results were such that experienced,
current pilots could discriminate more of what was said than
ex-pilots who in turn were able to discriminate more than
non-pilots. It is difficult to believe, on the basis of
masking, that these results have to do with some practiced
skill which allows you to perceive more of the signal in
noise. On the basis of my experience with such communication
systems, it is far more likely that the individuals most recently exposed to the communication format produced higher
scores simply on the basis of their greater familiarity with
the stilted pattern of the messages. In a second experiment,
normal hearing audiology graduate students demonstrated no
improvement in auditory discrimination in noise over extended
sessions (Birdwell, 1969). While their scores did not improve, it is interesting to note that each of them reported
less difficulty in understanding and less annoyance with the
interference as the series of sessions wore on. This increased confidence in performance and increased tolerance for
the obnoxious qualities of noise suggests that the hearing
aid wearer can improve his acceptance of communicating in
noise.

Although lipreading and amplification may provide the
bulk of the basis for rehabilitation, environmental controls
should form an explicit part of any curriculum. The hearing
impaired person should be made aware of several techniques
which are likely to improve his communication. The first is
to be sure that the person communicated with is aware of the
hearing loss. His understanding and tolerance certainly
contributes to efficient communication. Additionally, the.
person with a hearing loss should overcome a societal reticence about watching the speaker's face. He should come to
the understanding that it is alright to ask a person to offer

a view of his face so that he can better understand. I, for
example, have a habit of talking while using the blackboard,
thus displaying the back of my head for all to see. Class
members are encouraged to remind me to turn around while I am
talking. Other controls fall into two categories which
might best be summarized as keep it quiet and keep it close.
As I have become more aware of rehabilitation and as I have
grown older, I have come in social contact with a number of
households which include a hearing impaired individual. It
amazes me that, with only one exception, I find that a mur-
muring television or radio is an integral part of each house-
hold's operation. With the adverse effect of noise on communication there seems no excuse for an unattended babble in
the background. Noise reduction is an obvious way to improve
communication efficiency. It also amazes me to discover how
few people are aware of the practical effects of the inverse
square law. By halving the distance between communicators
it is possible to effect a 6 dB increase in the level of the
signal. Assuming the hearing impaired person is somewhere
on the rising portion of the articulation function, the simple expediency of halving the distance between communicators
can result in 20% improvement in a discrimination score.

   We have briefly discussed most of the major categories of information which should be made available to the
patient. It is time to turn to some of the mechanics of
putting a class together and pick up some categories of information that should be made available to both the patient
and those with whom he has daily contact, those who have been
termed "significant others".

   I have implied that group instruction should be pre-
ferable to individual. To prevent any misunderstanding, let
me make that explicit. With the exception of information
provided as part of the initial evaluation and the possible
follow-up visits associated with hearing aid fitting, I see
little value in dealing with rehabilitation on an individual
basis. There are obvious cases where it may be the only way
possible but you lose certain advantages of group instruction. Perhaps most importantly, in these days of cost
accounting, individual instruction costs more. In the interest of your individual good health, group instruction decreases the boredom of repetition by reducing the number of
cycles you go through in a given period of time. Group instruction provides a sheltered environment in with the patient can practice his developing communication skills with
people who have some sympathy for and understanding of hearing impairment.

I suggested earlier that it is important for the hearing impaired individual to make others aware of his hearing loss, particularly those with whom he has regular contact. As a novice to the careful analysis of hearing loss, he may be less than effective in transmitting the ramifications of his loss to significant others. For those others with whom he has the most constant and intimate contact, I advocate short circuiting their education by inviting them to the initial, if not all, class sessions. Two benefits accrue. First, their understanding can do much to alleviate the daily pressures of living with a hearing loss, freeing the patient to address his own rehabilitation. Secondly, a helpful partner can be valuable in implementing the practice necessary to eventual success in hearing aid use and lipreading. I emphasize that the initial sessions are important for both the patient and significant others. What is so important?

In essence and in a language suitable for the class members, the same material is covered that was reviewed for you when I discussed normal and abnormal hearing in the section on rationale. Not only should information be presented in a didactic menner but I have found it helpful for the normal hearing members of the class to listen to one of the records which approximate the effect of hearing loss. This is also an excellent time to stimulate candid discussions about the specific nature of communication problems encountered between the normal hearers and the hearing impaired. I have found it helpful to insure that the following topics be covered explicitly if not in response to spontaneous questions from the class:

1. The difference between awareness of an auditory event and discrimination of the nature of that event. Normal hearing individuals should be assured that it is possible for Grandpa to hear you talk while completely misunderstanding what you said and that the degree of understanding can vary as a function of noise, content and the rest of the factors which affect communication.

2. The effect of noise upon both normal understanding of speech and the aggravated effect of noise upon most hearing impaired individuals. It is stupid to talk to Grandpa with a radio playing progressive country rock.

3. The effect of distance upon the efficiency
of communication. It is stupid to try to talk
to Grandpa when he is in the bedroom and you
are in the kitchen, no matter how accustomed
you are to yelling at your kids.

While conducting such a class you had better be sure to review some of the exaggerations found in the popular literature. Someone is sure to ask the following questions:
1. Will acupuncture cure a hearing loss?

2. My friend had an operation whereby they
took a piece of a "nerve" from the back of
his hand and fixed his hearing. Why can't
I have the same operation?

3. How good are these nerve inplant techniques?

4. Is it really true that I can improve hearing
by changing my diet?

We have plowed through technique as if the patients
were motivated. I suggested that many of them are not and
promised to discuss some ways in which unmotivated patients
may be motivated. For these last few minutes let us categor-
ize patients as either living alone or with a few relatives
and those who may live in some larger group, such as a nursing home or a retirement community. Motivating the first
group is very close to impossible. If some relative has hog-
tied the patient long enough to undergo evaluation, it is
unlikely that he can be forced into some extended rehabilitation program. Assuming a need for rehabilitation and some
degree of cooperation on the part of the relative, the opportunity to motivate the patient can be had if issues such as
the use of one of those ugly hearing aids can be temporarily
skirted and both the patient and the relative can be induced
to attend the initial sessions of a rehabilitation class.
Better understanding of the capabilities and limitations of
those with hearing loss can certainly do no harm to the relative and, by proper emphasis on the capabilities, may encourage the hearing impaired person to continue the classes.
In effect the motivation is provided by the patient's understanding of possible improvement. Additional opportunities
are available for motivating the institutionalized patient.
Optional meetings which discuss hearing loss and its correction may prove to be the bait which will arouse the hearing
impaired individual's curiosity. An ongoing lipreading-

practice-social-club can provide the motivation to seek a
more structured, systematic approach to all deviating communication difficulties. For those who have a long history of
negative reward for attempting communication, one-on-one
visits where keep-it-close and keep-it-quiet rules are observed may begin the process of reestablishing positive reinforcement for communication. Nurses, volunteers and relatives are the ones who have to learn enough about communication with the hearing impaired to take the trouble to establish opportunities for the positive reinforcement. An
accessory which should be part of every institution which has
hearing impaired patients is one of the portable, battery
powered auditory training units for temporary use during
critical communication with those who have significant hearing impairments. An observable improvement during use of
amplification may be all that is necessary. It takes a stub-
born man to deny success.

A few moments ago I suggested that rehabilitation
could be motivated by bypassing hearing aid use. The broader
question of hearing aid use among the elderly needs to be
addressed. There are many factors which argue against hearing aid use. For those with mild losses, visual cues may be
enough to bring them into the range of effective communication. Hearing aids are expensive to obtain and maintain and
the elderly are likely to be past their income peak. Intelligent hearing aid use requires a degree of mental alertness
which may no longer be possible. When living alone there
may be only a small portion of time during which an aid is
required. The impact of hearing aid use upon the patient's
already deteriorating self-image may be more than his ego
can stand. For these and other reasons, demonstrable im-
provements in communication efficiency with amplification may
be ignored or side stepped. Alternatives to hearing aids
such as personal amplification for television, radio or telephone use may be effective for these activities. The combination of visual information, reasonable signal strength, low
levels of noise and the inescapable attention getting power
of being engaged by a human at close quarters, may override
the remaining limitations on communication.

That is aural rehabilitation, soup to nuts. You have
had nothing more than the broadest of overviews presented in
the most simplified way at the highest level of abstraction I
could muster. I have glossed over most of the pitfalls. I
can only hope that you have some context into which to structure the information that will follow.

REFERENCES

1. Berlin, C. I., Wexler, K. F., Jerger, J. F., Halperin,
    H. R. and Smith, S., Superior ultra-audiometric
    hearing: a new type of hearing loss which corre-
    lates highly with unusually good speech in the
    "profoundly deaf". *Otolaryngology, 86,* 111-116,
    1978.

2. Birdwell, P. B. The effect of practice on discrimina-
    tion in noise, Unpublished Thesis, Vanderbilt
    University, 1969.

3. Cooper, J. C. and Langley, L. R., Multiple choice speech
    discrimination tests for both diagnostic and rehab-
    ilitative evaluation: English and Spanish. *J. Acad.
    Rehab. Audiol., 11,* 132-141, 1978.

4. Gaeth, J., A study of phonemic regression in relation
    to hearing loss, Unpublished Dissertation, North-
    western University, 1948.

5. Gang, R. P. The effects of age on the diagnostic
    utility of the rollover phenomenon. *J. Spch. Hear.
    Dis., 41,* 63-69, 1976.

6. Unpublished Data., Audiology and Hearing Conservation
    Function, School of Aerospace Medicine, Brooks Air
    Force Base, Texas.

DISCUSSION

Audience: Can your panel address a total health care
team approach to aural rehabilitation? How would an audiologist fit in?
Deshayes: I like the team approach. I am on the
team at the University of Nebraska for Uniproach which deals
primarily with young children who have multiple problems. I
find a team approach very worthwhile because you get all the
disciplines involved working toward one goal and you do not
have to try to outguess or second guess somebody who is not
there. The whole team is there working together, planning
out a program for one particular person at a time. I like
this aspect to a team approach and I think this is possible
when working with the elderly, particularly where you are in
a nursing home setting. The nurses, the administrative personnel, everybody who is involved with that particular
person, should be on the team. If you miss one link, it
could mean failure for that particular patient.
Cooper: In your experience, who is the captain of
this team?
Deshayes: In Uniproach, we share the captainship.
For each patient, we choose a team leader and that person is
responsible for that particular patient. It is the team
leader's job to coordinate everything for the patient and
make sure that everything is done.
Cooper: Will you give us some of the professions
associated with the team?
Deshayes: On ours we have a speech pathologist, an
audiologist, a social worker, psychiatrist, a neurologist,
psychoneurologist, and a pediatrician.
Cooper: Dr Henoch, your comments on the team
approach.
Henoch: I think in terms of work with the elderly,
especially in nursing home environments, that it is vitally
important to utilize the team approach. I think the audiologist who is engaged in aural rehabilitation in that kind of
a setting is going to need the additional information in
order to be able to work with the patient. You need the kind
of input that the social worker, psychologist or nurse who
works closely with the patient can give to you. You cannot
jump in knowing nothing about the individual. The team
approach is absolutely necessary in a nursing home setting.

Audience: Now you keep mentioning nursing homes. I think most of us know that less than 5% of the elderly population lives in a nursing home. I think maybe we are addressing ourselves too much to a small population. The well elderly in the community have to be looked at in a different way when dealing with them through a team approach.

Henoch: I agree with that. The question is, where are you gathering these people together? A senior citizen's center is one place where you could have this kind of thing. I can see using the team approach in that setting. In a university clinic, if you have something similar to our Center for Studies on Aging, all of the team members would be available to you. There is no reason why, if a program is conducted in a senior citizen center, these people could not be utilized as part of the team.

Audience: I would like to address the question. I have been working in a senior citizen retirement apartment community. I feel that this is where you find the bulk of the seniors. In this setting our team has been the audiologist, the activities director, who may be a resident of the facility, and the resident manager. That has worked well. I think if we try to exclude anybody, we are in trouble.

Deshayes: Talking about the team for the elderly outside the nursing home, I have found, particularly in Nebraska and in Lincoln where I am, a very important team member is the minister. Lincoln is unique in that we have 190,000 people and 260 churches. So we have more churches per 1,000 people than any other city in the United States. Ministers are very involved and I have found that most of them are quite concerned about hearing problems and work very well with the hearing impaired. This is important because they are the ones that will get into the homes and they are the ones that are always at our meetings to learn about rehabilitation problems. One of their big concerns is what they can do to make their churches a better place to hear.

Cooper: If a person is coordinating inservice training in a care center it would seem that the coordinator might have some comments about team efforts and how you get the team effort into the program on a day to day basis. I would be interested in hearing comments from someone like that.

Darlene Lacey: I work in a nursing home. We have a physician who works very closely with us and he is tremendous. I think this has probably been our biggest asset. We have had a tremendous problem in our community with getting

involvement from outside of the medical profession. We have
a speech therapist that will work with us but she is not
associated with the facility. I am an RN. My director, the
doctor, and I have done most of the teamwork because we are
having so much trouble getting anyone from the speech and
audiology fields to come into the facility.

Chapter 4

Development, Composition and
Problems with Elderly Aural
Rehabilitation Groups

HARRIET KAPLAN, PH. D.

INTRODUCTION

Today I would like to talk about an aural rehabilitation program that I and colleagues in the Washington D.C.
area have used in a number of different settings. Although
we have used it with younger adults as well as geriatrics,
for our purposes I will restrict the discussion to two senior
citizen populations: elderly clients living independently in
retirement apartment communities and geriatrics in nursing
homes. First I would like to describe the program and then
follow with a discussion of strengths, weaknesses, and issues
that we need to deal with.

THE POPULATION

It is important to understand that in the retirement
apartment community and in the nursing home we are dealing
with different populations, although there is overlap. Since
differences do exist, a program must be modified appropriately for the two situations. Typically the retirement apartment community consists of separate living units which the
older individuals or couples manage themselves. They meet
their own everyday living needs, manage their own financial
affairs, and come and go as they like. There is almost
always a resident manager who serves as big brother, sympathetic ear, helper, friend as well as property manager. In
many situations there is a program director who may be a
senior citizen resident of the house. Other facilities hire
professional activities directors. In most situations there
is a communal dining arrangement for lunch and dinner which
is optional but generally very popular with the residents.
Mealtimes are major social events but seem to be one of the
most difficult communicative situations. Although people
living in these retirement communities often have multiple

physical problems, they do not need skilled nursing care;
they function independently, some with slight assistance.
Most of these apartments are either low or moderate income
dwellings, although there are some privately developed communities for the more affluent senior citizens. Still most
of the independently living elderly are under some financial
constraints.

       The nursing home population is generally older, more
physically disabled, and shows a higher incidence of organic
brain syndrome. The residents there are dependent on nursing
home personnel to meet their physical, social, and emotional
needs. Usually they lack financial independence. The typical nursing home resident pays the cost of his maintenance
through his social security or other pension income from
which the nursing home administrator sets aside a small personal allowance. So long as the resident lives in the nursing home, he experiences limited ability to make financial
decisions or other decisions about matters of daily living.
He infrequently leaves the home for recreational purposes and
must be content with activities that are provided by the
home.

       In terms of physical and mental capabilities, there
is overlap between the retirement community and the nursing
home. There are many alert senior citizens who choose to
enter nursing homes even though they do not need skilled nursing care or even intermediate care. In some cases, this decision is a form of insurance that a place in the nursing
home of choice will be available when needed.

DESCRIPTION OF THE PROBLEM

       The program consists of both assessment and rehabili-
tative procedures. Rehabilitation consists primarily of
group instruction in speechreading and auditory training as
well as educational counseling regarding nature of hearing
loss, advantages and disadvantages of amplification, and ways
of managing difficult communication situations. While the
classes are in progress, individual speechreading and/or
auditory training may be taking place. In addition, pure
tone testing with subsequent counseling or simply counseling
by itself may be occurring.

ASSESSMENT PROCEDURES
  Threshold Tests

       Assessment procedures are initiated with air and bone
conduction threshold testing conducted in a quiet room in the

center where the program is held. Individual interviews take
place at the same time. The threshold tests have two purposes: (1) to identify anyone who might need medical evaluation as evidenced by the presence of air-bone gaps; (2) to
identify those people who seem to be candidates for hearing
aids. In either case, clients are referred either to the
audiology clinic associated with the program or another
approved facility. When necessary, transportation is
arranged for or provided by those conducting the program.

Interview

        The interview procedure is designed to reveal infor-
mation about probable cause of the hearing problem, existing
contributory medical problems, difficult communication situations, what the client hopes to achieve in the program, what
his motivation is with regard to amplification, and his feelings about himself as a hearing impaired person. The interview, which is conducted at the same time as the audiometric
testing, is also designed to develop rapport and trust between client and audiologist. It is vital that the senior
citizen feel that the clinician is genuinely interested in
him as an individual; the groundwork for the therapeutic relationship is laid during the interview.

REHABILITATION PROCEDURES
Hearing Aid Evaluations

        Hearing aid evaluations are normally performed in the
audiology clinic. However, for those unable to travel, informal assessments and fittings have been conducted in the
clinets' homes. When a hearing aid is recommended for a participant in the program, ongoing follow-up and hearing aid
orientation are conducted on a weekly basis for as long as is
necessary. The presence of the audiologist in the center
each week makes this very easy.
        Ideally, a recommended hearing aid should be a new
instrument, selected for that particular client. However,
funding is often a problem, and since in most cases third
party payments are not available, we must sometimes settle
for used hearing aids. In such cases, the audiologist must
assure that these instruments are functioning acceptably in
terms of electroacoustic characteristics.
        Whenever a hearing aid is recommended, a trial period
is always arranged and closely supervised. Sometimes a
client is permitted to use the clinic model of the recommended hearing aid during therapy for several weeks before final

recommendation of the aid. Sometimes a client experiments
with several settings or instruments during therapy before a
final decision is made. All hearing aids which are purchased
come with at least a 30 day home trial.

Speechreading

        A portion of all meetings is devoted to speechreading
practice. Although I do not know how much speechreading
training has improved overall communication, subjectively I
am aware that group members have generally become more visually attentive. After a period of therapy there is increased
willingness to attend to the face of the speaker and to use
contextual and situational clues to a greater extent. Interestingly enough, the majority of clients upon entering the
program indicate that they do not look at people's faces when
communicating with them. Regardless of the contribution
speechreading makes to overall communication, senior citizens
consider it their primary goal. For that reason, it is an
integral part of every lesson. Speechreading therapy is primarily synthetic in nature, including work on homophenes,
idiomatic expressions, dialogues, etc. Much emphasis is
placed on the use of linguistic and situational redundancy
inherent in our language. Therapists are free to select any
techniques and materials they feel are appropriate for their
clients but the fundamental principle is that all materials
must be relevant to the life situations of the group
members.

Auditory Training

        Auditory training includes the following: (a) prac-
tice sessions to aid the clients in adjusting to reduced or
distorted auditory signals; (b) training in improving habits
of auditory attentiveness; (c) illustration of environmental
manipulation to maximize use of audition. For example, many
clients do not realize that they can hear a speaker far better if the good ear, aided or not, is facing the speaker.
Similarly, it is not apparent to many hearing impaired people
that understanding in noise is easier if both listener and
speaker move themselves as far away from the noise source as
possible. These are examples of instruction in environmental
manipulation. Auditory training with the group is synthetic,
often using the same materials as the speechreading part of
the lesson. It can be performed in quiet, against competing
noise or competing speech, live voice or using taped materials. We try to simulate life situations as much as possible.

Discussion and Counseling

A lecture-discussion is a part of each session. Topics include: (1) explanation of hearing and hearing loss,
(2) adjustment and communicative problems attributable to
hearing loss and techniques for managing communication situations, (3) advantages and disadvantages of hearing aids, (4)
hearing aid use and care, (5) telephone, television, and
other listening aids, (6) consumerism. Both informational
and personal adjustment counseling occur through these sessions. In the discussion of difficult listening situations,
a certain amount of assertiveness training is incorporated.
Those problem situations identified during the initial interviews are discussed and suggestions for assertive handling of
these situations are elicited from the group. Sometimes the
therapists role play such situations. For all discussions
visual aids are used as much as possible.

Several sessions are usually devoted to discussion of
hearing aids: what they are, how they work, what they will
and will not do, what goes on during a hearing aid evaluation, use and care of the aid. These sessions usually follow
other lectures on nature of hearing loss and difficult listening situations. Many people become interested in trying
hearing aids only after such sessions.

An important goal of aural rehabilitation is acceptance of one's hearing loss and the ability to accept oneself
as a hearing impaired person. One way to facilitate this
goal is to encourage consumerism among the hearing impaired
themselves. The problems of the hearing impaired in obtaining services from the community are very real. For example,
in the Washington D.C. area smoke detectors are mandatory in
all households but there is no smoke detector on the market
that has a visual warning signal. Thus the hearing impaired
person is forced to install useless gadgets in his or her
home. In order to remedy such problems and to increase
acceptance of themselves as hearing impaired persons, we encourage activism among our clients. I do not recommend activism in the nursing home, however, even though it has
worked well in the retirement apartment communities and senior citizen clubs. In the nursing home, residents vent their
anger on the administration, with unfortunate results for the
program.

Inservice Training

In the nursing home inservice training of nursing
aides, volunteers, office staff, and perhaps nursing staff is

essential. This is the one aspect of aural rehabilitation
that most nursing home administrators find valuable, although
many are not receptive to other aspects of a program. Since
the nursing home aide has the greatest amount of contact with
the hearing impaired resident, inservice training should be
geared to his level of understanding. It should focus on two
areas: the use and care of hearing aids and how to talk to
hearing impaired people. I have found that two or three one
hour training sessions are sufficient for a group. Since
there is considerable turnover of personnel in nursing homes,
however, these in-service training sessions need to be repeated frequently. It is well to use visual aids, particularly in the discussions of hearing aids, and allow some
hands-on experience to demonstrate that aids do not "disinte-
grate" or "blow up" when handled.

        In many nursing homes donated used aids or instru-
ments belonging to deceased residents are given to other residents either as primary hearing aids or as loaners. Generally these hearing aids are in various states of disrepair
and the person responsible for dispensing them is either a
volunteer or a member of the office staff. Generally this
individual knows very little about hearing aids or differences in amplification needs of hearing impaired people. A
resident in need of a hearing aid is simply given any instrument that happens to work. The audiologist can perform a
valuable service by testing these instruments electroacousti-
cally, eliminating those that are not functioning adequately,
classifying the others as to appropriate gain, SSPL, and frequency response, and instructing the people in charge for
what type of loss each aid is suitable.

        In addition to information about hearing aids, nurs-
ing home personnel need information about earmolds. They
need to understand the importance of proper fit, what causes
feedback, how to help residents insert molds properly, and
routine cleaning and care.

Peer Counseling

        In the non-institutionalized setting, we are con-
cerned with peer counseling rather than in-service training.
In order to minimize communication difficulties for the hearing impaired, it is important that the people with whom they
live understand the problems associated with hearing loss.
In the apartment communities these people are the neighbors
of our clients. The information shared with them is essentially the same as that which is discussed during in-service
training sessions at the nursing home.

We have attempted to reach non-group members in a
number of ways. First, all group members have been encouraged to bring friends to class. These friends may have hearing losses themselves or have normal hearing. Clients have
been almost evangelistic in recruiting their neighbors and a
number of these recruits have subsequently become clients
themselves. Similar invitations have been extended to families of residents.

Second, we consistently have advertised our program
within the facility in which it is being held. This has
been done through regular announcements in the dining hall
and at residents' meetings. At least once a year I have
spoken to the residents at one of their meetings. People
have been informed of the various services available to
them, such as audiometric testing and individual counseling,
in addition to the aural rehabilitation classes. Many people who have not joined the classes have taken advantage of
the testing and counseling services.

Still another way of reaching peers is to use the
weekly or monthly newspaper that is printed in most retirement apartments and in many nursing homes. We have made it a
a point to submit something to each issue, either suggestions on how to speak to a hearing impaired person, tips
about handling difficult listening situations, or information
about use and care of hearing aids.

I have found that the peer counseling has been perhaps the most successful part of the aural rehabilitation
program. Through it, we have been able to reach far more
people than those who have actually attended classes on a
continuing basis.

Issues

For the remainder of this session I would like to
talk about various issues that relate to the development and
management of aural rehabilitation programs. We have managed to resolve some problems but others are unsolved. Perhaps you have found answers where we have not.

Motivation

One question that is asked frequently is "How do you
motivate senior citizens to come for therapy?" I think we
need to look at the motivation issue on two levels.

First, there is a need to motivate key professionals
in the senior citizen facilities in which we wish to work.
It is important that administrators, social workers, and

activities directors fully accept our programs and make a
commitment to work with us. In one apartment building, the
manager was not fully committed to our program. Consequently, she did not make an effort to inform and interest the
residents. As a result, people did not attend class. Unless
a key person in the facility is convinced of the merits of
the program, success is improbable. In the retirement communities the key person is usually the resident manager; in
the senior citizen center it is usually a social worker or an
activities director; in the nursing home one must approach
the administrator of the facility. It is necessary to explain the program in a face-to-face meeting and also leave
written material. I have found apartment managers and social
workers in senior citizen centers very receptive when the
benefits of the program were clearly explained.

We have had less success with nursing home administrators in our community. I do not know if this is simply
the situation in the Washington D.C. area, or if it reflects
a national trend. We have found that some administrators did
not even wish to discuss aural rehabilitation programs.
Others were receptive to inservice training but nothing else.
In some cases audiometric screening was permitted but there
was no follow-up. A bit of probing revealed that some administrators tended to confuse us with hearing aid dealers and
feared that their residents would be exploited or that eventually our program would cost the nursing home money. This
tendency to confuse us with the hearing aid industry and the
fear of exploitation can only be overcome through community
education. We need to use the media and obtain the support
of community leaders including representatives of local government. This type of public relations work is time consuming but very necessary. Unfortunately I have not been able
to do enough of this.

The fear of some nursing home administrators that an
aural rehabilitation program will cost the home money is
sometimes justified. I would like to tell you about an aural
rehabilitation program in a nursing home that was unsuccessful because of this problem. The home was a well run church
oriented facility which employed a full time social worker
who arranged a variety of activities for the residents. The
administrator was dedicated to the people in his charge. We
had been asked by the social worker to develop a program in
the home; she was extremely helpful in providing physical
facilities and making sure the residents came to class on
time. Interest among the residents was high, especially
among those people who were in reasonably good health.
Things went well until a number of the residents became

interested in trying hearing aids. Although the interest in
amplification was there, the funding was not, since medicare
does not cover hearing aid costs. Since in an institution
the administrator controls all aspects of a resident's life,
including the financial, our clients expected him to provide
money for hearing aids. At the end of the semester, we were
invited to take our program elsewhere. We had created a desire for better hearing among the residents but in doing so
had inadvertantly created a threatening situation for the
administration.

In the independent living units, each person controls
his own financial situation, and either can produce funding
for amplification or must continue without it. Although financial contingencies exist in both environments, they do
not impact the non-institutional program in the same way.

The second level of motivation concerns the senior
citizen clients themselves. There is indeed a motivation
problem, which I feel is related to attitudes about themselves as hearing impaired people. When an individual joins
an aural rehabilitation group or even requests a test, he
implicitly acknowledges that he has a hearing problem and
wants to do something about it. Many hearing impaired people, including seniors, deny the reality of the hearing loss,
perhaps because it is a tangible indication of the aging
process. Other elderly people just give up; they feel there
is nothing worth hearing, that their lives lack meaning, that
they are too old to learn. This attitude is far more preva-
lent in the nursing home than in the apartment community.

There is no magic cure for denial and depression; we
cannot suddenly create changes in feelings. What we can do
is inform all residents of a facility that we are interested
in them, are available to help whenever they are ready, and
are willing to accept them on their terms. It must be made
clear that they are welcome to sample a few lessons or simply
come in to talk with the audiologist. Use of amplification
is not a prerequisite for participation in the program. It
is important to interact with the people in the facility a
bit outside of class, perhaps only with a few friendly words
in the lobby. By working with those people who are ready to
make a commitment and by engaging in as many peer counseling
activities as possible, eventually we reach some of the un-
committed. What we try to do is create the attitude that it
is acceptable to have a hearing problem and that one can live
productively in spite of it. I'm sure Dr. Alpiner will say
much more about psychological and social factors tomorrow.

In the retirement apartments as well as in the nursing homes there was sometimes suspicion of our motives. In

almost all of the programs it took months to convince the
residents that we were not interested in merely selling them
hearing aids. For this reason and because I firmly believe
that hearing impaired people, particularly senior citizens,
must be strongly motivated to use amplification to be successful with it, hearing aid evaluation was not stressed at
the beginning of the program. It was made very clear to all
participants that one does not have to use a hearing aid to
benefit from the program; that if and when an individual
feels the need for amplification we would help him select an
appropriate instrument. In most cases, little hearing aid
evaluation work occurred during the first semester of
therapy.

In all the facilities in which we have worked, atten-
dance at the first meeting was very good, provided the person
in charge of the center was supportive. People were curious
to see what we were offering. The amount of attrition that
followed during subsequent classes depended primarily on how
well we met needs. We learned that since people attend
classes for as long as they feel they are benefiting from the
experience, we had to be constantly attuned to their needs.
It was necessary to be flexible in preparing lessons and to
shift gears when necessary. Often questions asked during a
discussion determined the nature of the following discussion
although originally some other topic was scheduled at that
time. Sometimes a discussion became so productive that
speechreading or auditory training was not conducted at that
session.

The needs of the clients influenced lesson planning
in other ways. All materials used for speechreading and
auditory training had to be relevant to the clients' life
situations. All clients had to experience success each week,
since apparent lack of progress would invariably lead to
withdrawal from class. In order to insure success for each
person each week, it was necessary to individualize presentation of material so that everyone functioned at the proper
level. Proper individualization of material required careful
planning since the groups were heterogeneous. If someone
required individual counseling on a particular day, he was
removed from class to receive that counseling. Generally, we
found that in these ways we could maintain fairly stable
classes of approximately ten people.

Sometimes clients did not come to class because they
forgot, despite constant reminders. Short memory span is a
very real problem with this population. On more than one
occasion we have gone to a person's apartment or room to remind him that class was in session. We have also requested

that weekly announcements be made at dinner the night before class to remind people of aural rehabilitation the following day.

In short, those clients who have made a commitment to improve their communication will attend class on a regular basis as long as they feel they are benefiting from the experience. Our job is to try to meet their needs as best as we can.

Physical Arrangements - Transportation

Senior citizens typically have transportation problems, regardless of the environments in which they live. These are caused by limited public transportation, physical problems which make the use of public transportation difficult, limited funds for taxicabs, and fear of crime or of exploring the unknown. For all these reasons, it is unrealistic to expect the elderly client to come to a clinic for aural rehabilitation. We must bring our programs to them. In each place we have worked, we have arranged to conduct our program in a specific place in the building for two hours each week. Personnel, materials, and equipment were all transported to the senior citizen facility. Generally, room space was not a problem, although it was occasionally necessary to search through the building a bit to find a room with reasonable acoustics and lighting.

Two aspects of the program that could not be performed at the senior citizen center were hearing aid evaluations and follow-up testing to explore the nature of air-bone gaps. Transportation to the clinic had to be handled on an individual basis. Sometimes children would transport their parents but in most cases the senior citizens were adamant about maintaining independence. In some cases a resident of the apartment building with a car would transport others. Volunteer organizations in the community were sometimes used but were found to be of questionable reliability. In many cases we provided transportation in our own cars. In one way or another those people who needed to visit the campus clinic managed to get there, but we found that we had to assume the responsibility of making arrangements more often than we preferred.

Visiting the doctor or the hearing aid dealer presented the same kind of transportation difficulty, particularly in the nursing home. In some nursing homes, however, physicians made regular calls or were available at all times. This practice alleviated some of the transportation difficulties. Hearing aid dealers however were generally not welcome

in senior citizen facilities. It would help considerably if
an audiologist-sponsored dealer could arrange to make regular
visits to senior citizen residences, or if the audiologist
were to "dispense" within the senior citizen facility.
    Another form of transportation difficulty is encoun-
tered primarily in the nursing home. Some of the clients may
be in wheelchairs or for other reasons be unable to get to
class without help. Since it is impractical for the audiologist to physically dress, brace, and wheel clients to
class, this kind of support must be negotiated with the social worker, activities director or whomever the appropriate
person may be. If the management is supportive of the program, this will not be a problem. If, however, the audiologist is required to prepare and transport clients to class,
the success of the program is doubtful.

Scheduling

    It is important to schedule classes at times that do
not conflict with other happenings in the facility such as
meal times, physical therapy, ceramics classes, etc. In
order to find an optimal time for the program it is important
to work with the activities director or the social worker.
Once a class time has been scheduled, it should not be
changed unless absolutely necessary. Older people tend to be
creatures of habit and once they have learned to expect a
class at a certain time, change is very difficult. In one
facility we conducted our classes on Friday morning for a
year and then had to change to Monday morning to avoid a
scheduling conflict. Despite constant reminders, it took
three months for all members of our group to stop coming to
class on Friday morning.
    We are all accustomed to performing audiological
evaluation first, and then developing therapy programs based
on the test data. When I first started geriatric aural rehabilitation, I made it a point to complete all diagnostics
before starting therapy, since this is a logical procedure.
By the time I got around to rehabilitation, however, my
clients had vanished.. In the two or three weeks needed for
evaluation, they had become disenchanted with the program
because therapy was not being offered. From this experience
I learned that therapy must begin immediately and that testing should be performed concurrently. Generally, by the end
of the third week we have interview and audiological data on
most of our group members.

Personnel

The clinicians for all of my programs have been graduate students. I have found this arrangement desirable for
a number of reasons. First, aural rehabilitation activity
provides excellent training for students. Skills in speechreading and auditory training techniques which are developed
can be used with younger adults and older children as well
as senior citizens. Much of the educational counseling which
the students perform can be adapted to parent groups. Valuable training in group therapy techniques, particularly in
individualization of presentation of material is provided.

Second, elderly people tend to relate well to young
people interested in their problems and are very flattered
that students wish to work with them. Since there is a pre-
ponderance of females in the senior citizen groups, male
therapists are especially appreciated. Last semester I
brought a male therapist into one of my groups composed
largely of women. That young man found himself with at
least a dozen adopted grandmothers who provided ample sup-
plies of cookies, cake and other treats.

Third, students can serve as extensions of the audiologist, and allow for increased program flexibility. I have
always used two students in each program to perform team
therapy with the clients in a group situation, allowing the
use of techniques such as skits, dialogues, etc. In addition, I have often simultaneously assigned a third student
therapist to work with an individual or a small group in need
of intensive speechreading or auditory training work. Occasionally, a fourth student has been recruited for pure tone
testing. While all this is going on, the supervisor is free
to observe the work of the groups, participate where necessary, or counsel an individual client. Since it is difficult
to commit that number of trained professionals to a single
program, students meet the need very well.

Of course, students must be properly trained and
supervised, but this does not need to be an insurmountable
problem. I require the following prerequisite knowledge and
skills of all student clinicians in the senior citizen programs: (1) academic work in basic audiological testing,
audiometric interpretation, hearing aid orientation and trou-
bleshooting, and techniques of aural rehabilitation; and (2)
previous practicum experience with adults so that the student
can relate to clients in a therapy situation. Conceivably
without these prerequisites, a student's performance could be
less than optimal. The students are given guidelines as to
the nature and direction of the program. They are required

to submit weekly lesson plans and meet with the supervisor
regularly. This arrangement can be developed in a hospital
or community clinic as well as in a university if the clinic
is interested in serving as a practicum affiliation for a
university training program.

Hearing Aids

        Although Dr. Kasten will discuss at length evaluation
and fitting of hearing aids, I would like to share with you
a few of my observations regarding amplification with this
population. Of those senior citizens who seemed to be good
hearing aid candidates in terms of type of loss, discrimination ability and motivation, a significant number, perhaps
30 to 40 percent, returned their instruments during the trial
period. In most cases motivation and fit of the hearing aid
seemed adequate, and in all cases hearing aid orientation
preceded and followed the purchase of the aid. I believe
there is much we do not know about the nature and effects of
presbycusis and with the present state of the art cannot
accurately predict who is and who is not a good hearing aid
candidate. Until our predictive abilities improve, our
clients must be assured that they will not lose their money
should the hearing aid experiment not be successful, that an
aid can be returned to the dealer during the trial period
with full refund guaranteed. They should also be made to
understand that failure with amplification does not indicate
any kind of personal inadequacy, nor does it disqualify them
from the aural rehabilitation program.
        Earlier in this discussion I alluded to the problems
caused by lack of adequate funding. Money for repair of
used instruments is sometimes just as hard to find as money
for purchase of new hearing aids. Yet, if we must rely on
used instruments we must make sure they are in good working
condition. I have performed electroacoustic testing on a
fair number of donated hearing aids and have found extremely
high levels of distortion. Sometimes charitable groups in
the community such as the Lions Club or Sertoma can be called
upon to donate repair money. In some situations hearing aid
dealers can be induced to consider such repairs charitable
contributions useful as tax deductions. Sometimes a client
himself can afford to repair a used aid but not to purchase a
new one. If the audiologist cannot find a way to have a malfunctioning instrument repaired, he should discard it.

Composition of the Senior Citizen Group

First, let us talk about who is eligible for the program. In my opinion, there are no good audiological criteria
to determine which elderly people need aural rehabilitation.
The majority of residents of any senior citizen community
show pure tone thresholds poorer than 25 dB HL, yet not all
have communication difficulties. We could use the presbycusis curves based on the American Standards Association
data[1,2], accepting only those people who deviate in sensitivity from the norms for their age. However, this criterion
does not give us a valid indication of how much communicative difficulty an individual is experiencing. Speechreading
tests provide a measure of how well an individual can understand unrelated sentences under a given set of testing conditions, but they do not tell us much about overall communication difficulties or adjustment to hearing impairment. I
believe that any individual who feels he can benefit from an
aural rehabilitation program should be encouraged to enter
one, regardless of degree or type of loss.

There are certain exceptions to the "open enrollment"
that I am proposing. Since a major component of an aural
rehabilitation program is speechreading training, blind individuals obviously would experience much frustration. In
one of the nursing homes in which we developed a program, an
overzealous social worker enrolled several totally blind
hearing impaired people into the group, despite discourage-
ment from the audiologist. The experience proved quite frustrating to these people who dropped out of the program after
two or three sessions. We subsequently formed a special
group for the blind people in which the emphasis was hearing
aid orientation, auditory training, and educational counseling. Partially sighted people, as opposed to blind, can
frequently fit nicely into a heterogeneous group so long as
their vision is adequate to clearly see the face of the
speaker. If such individuals become part of a group, certain
modifications must be made. Extra attention must be paid to
lighting and seating, and large bold print must be used for
anything written on paper or a blackboard.

People who are suffering from senility or severe emotional problems are likewise poor candidates for an aural
rehabilitation group. If time and personnel permit, however,
these people can be worked with individually or in small
groups with the emphasis placed on communication strategies
that work best for them. For these people manipulation of
the environment, particularly education of caregivers, may be
the most important part of therapy.

When should a person be dismissed from an aural rehabilitation group? With the current state of the art, there is no evaluative tool to inform us when a given individual has received maximum benefit from the program. We have experimented with communication scales such as the Denver Scale[3] and the Hearing Handicap Scale[4], primarily for the purpose of evaluating progress. We have found that although these scales have provided insight into the nature of the individual's communication problems, they have not proved to be optimal tools for evaluating progress. With most of our clients, we have found the pencil-and-paper test impossible because of visual problems, short attention span, and lack of understanding of items. We have found the concept of the semantic differential very difficult for many of these people who, despite heroic attempts on the part of the examiners, tend to give yes-no responses to questions. We have also found poor test-retest reliability with a majority of clients. I have found that each individual decides for himself when he is ready to leave the group. Members are encouraged to continue attending sessions for as long as they feel their communication is improving. Our programs have continued in a given setting for as long as interest has been maintained.

Although we would like to work with homogeneous groups, heterogeniety is the more realistic condition. For the speechreading aspect of the program the heterogeneity does not pose a serious problem since presentation of material can be individualized. From time to time new arrivals in a group have expressed frustration because their skills were obviously inferior to those of people who had participated in the program longer. These newcomers were worked with individually until they "caught up".

Since a group may contain members who had participated the previous semester as well as new arrivals, initially we were concerned about the repetitiveness of the lecture-discussion material for long-term group members. We found, however, that a certain amount of forgetting occurred from one semester to another and consequently repetition was welcome. In addition, discussions were modified from semester to semester. For example, some of our most useful discussions dealt with explanations of audiograms of group members in terms of how test results relate to communication problems. Each time new people entered the group, there were new audiograms and different communication problems to discuss.

The heterogeneity of the groups has impacted auditory training procedures. Although all auditory training has been synthetic and has used material relevant to common life

situations of the clients, individualizing presentation has
been difficult. Some clients with severe hearing losses have
required audiovisual presentation while others have not been
stressed sufficiently with this type of input. When competing signal is used, different signal-to-noise ratios are
needed for each person and for each type of material. Constant experimentation and adjustment of noise levels are
necessary. If anyone in the group has a tolerance problem,
that person may not be able to tolerate levels of noise
necessary for others in the group. Although we continue to
experiment with synthetic auditory training with our heterogeneous groups, we have been more successful when working
with individuals or with small homogeneous groups.

Conclusions

I have found geriatric aural rehabilitation dynamic
and exciting. Once initial suspicions are overcome, the
clients are appreciative and eager to learn. We have much to
offer these people and much to learn from them. Despite the
many problems, I consider the efforts to be most worthwhile.

REFERENCES

1. American Standards Association Subcommittee X24-X2
    Report: The Relations of Hearing Loss to Noise
    Exposure, New York: American Standards Association,
    1954.

2. Glorig, A., D. Wheeler, R. Quiggle, W. Grings, and
    A. Summerfield, 1954 Wisconsin State Fair Hearing
    Survey., Monograph, American Academy of Ophthalmology
    and Otolaryngology, 1957.

3. Alpiner, J. G., W. Chevrette, M. Metz, B. Olsen, The
    Denver Scale of Communication Function, Unpublished
    study, University of Denver, 1974.

4. High, W., G. Fairbanks, and A. Glorig., Scale for self-
    assessment of hearing handicap. J. Speech and
    Hearing Disorders, 29, 215-230, 1964.

Chapter 5

Evaluation and Fitting of
Amplification for the
Aging Population

ROGER E. KASTEN, PH. D.

Our task today is to speak about the evaluation and
fitting of amplification systems to the hearing impaired
aging population. I would wish that we could provide a
rather direct and simplified model for the task at hand. I
would refer particularly to the model presented by Frankel
(1972) for the eradication of poverty. While the eradication
of poverty may seem difficult, Frankel has presented a detailed model that gives us a straight line function for this
complex task. According to Frankel's model, before individuals had money there was poverty, after the acquisition of
money, there was no poverty. Notice how cleverly he deals
with the essential information. Why can't we provide a model
as easy as this when dealing with the many complexities of
communicatively impaired aging population?
    Indeed, Botwinick (1973) has pointed out that older
individuals are frequently withdrawn and introverted. He has
also indicated that they seem to be overly cautious, more
prone to depression and generally rigid. Cumming and Henry
(1961) have stated that the older individual is frequently
more preoccupied with self rather than with the environment
surrounding self. Gilbert and Levee (1971) have indicated
that a characteristic of the aging population is a decline in
both short-term and long-term memory span. In short, our
dealings with the auditory rehabilitation of the aging population brings us face to face with a complex group of individuals who possess both a unique set of capabilities and a
seemingly almost preordained set of disabilities.
    When we talk about the evaluation or fitting of am-
plification systems to the aging population we are constantly
dealing with a nomenclature nonentity. We are not dealing
with a single population, but rather we are dealing with at
least three separate populations. These populations are
separate in terms of life style, but frequently they are not
altogether too separate in terms of life ability. Specifically, we are dealing with the independent living aging

population, the semi-independent population and the dependent
living aging population.

As we look first at the independent living population, we immediately realize that this, in itself, is not a
single entity. Chatfield (1977) has pointed out, using the
Life Satisfaction Index, that aging individuals not surpris-
ingly use their yearly income as a significant means of
establishing their own individual degree of lifetime satisfaction. Chatfield also points out that the independent
living aging individuals use their location for living as a
crucial determinant of overall satisfaction, with those
living in a family unit being significantly more satisfied
than those not living in a family. As we come face to face
with the independent living aging individual, we must realize
that we are dealing with a complex individual. This is a
person, regardless of whether they are male or female, who
has lived out their conventionally productive life and now
views their own future with varying degrees of optimism or
pessimism. Indeed, with this population, the desire to play
a productive role in future interpersonal activities is
critical toward their prognosis for communicative success.

All of us have, at one time or another, come in contact with the independent living aging individual who sees
absolutely no need for continued success in communicative
situations and can find no benefit from improvement in the
communicative environment. These are the individuals that we
classify as having a poor degree of motivation. The factors
leading to this attitude are often many and varied. Loether
(1975), quoting the Special Committee on Aging of the United
States Senate, points out that the aging population are prime
candidates for the dealings of unscrupulous hearing aid
salesmen. Loether is not alone in this sentiment since the
RPAG report (1973), and the Minnesota report (1972), voiced
essentially the same theme. If we couple these findings with
the general statement heard from many older individuals that
they are not interested in amplification since most of their
friends have not received help from amplification, the individual outlook on the part of the aging individual for high
motivation is not overly encouraging.

As we approach the evaluation process, it must be
accomplished with a high degree of optimism. This is not to
indicate that we should tell the aging individual that an
amplification system is going to remove all of their problems, but we must make it clear that a properly fitted amplification system can alleviate many of the communicatively
negative situations that aging individuals face. Indeed, the
independent living aging individual must be made to realize

that an amplification device will provide help in the more
favorable listening situations and will provide sound in the
more unfavorable listening situations. The total evaluative
process for the aging independently living individual will
not be altogether unlike the evaluative process used with any
other adult. Particular care must be taken to insure that
the aging individual does not fatigue during the process of
the evaluation. Botwinick (1973) has pointed out that a
rather rapid fatigue process is characteristic of the aging
population. Care must be taken to insure that the results of
the evaluative process are not contaminated and unduly affected by fatigue as opposed to reaction to amplification
systems.

Fatigue, however, is not the only factor that must be
considered. Kasten and Thomas (1978) examined the speech
discrimination ability of a group of individuals over the age
of 70. All subjects used in this investigation yielded
intelligibility scores of between 35% and 85% on a conventional speech discrimination measurement. The investigators
then presented to the subjects a predetermined "correct-
incorrect" indication by means of two differently colored
lights. In one condition the subject received an indication
of an 85% correct rate regardless of the actual level of
their performance. In another condition, they received an
indication of a 35% correct rate regardless of their actual
level of performance. Interestingly, under both conditions,
one thought to create positive feedback and the other thought
to create negative feedback, the actual intelligibility performance of the aging individuals increased markedly.
Indeed, under either reinforcement scheme, a mean improvement
of approximately 28% was found over the performance achieved
in the conventional measurement scheme. It was felt by
Kasten and Thomas that the improvement resulted from an increase in interest, an increase in motivation, an increase in
attention, an increase in effort, or some combination of
these factors brought about by the reinforcement feedback
scheme used in the investigation.

As a result, it is important to keep in mind that,
with this population, the investigators were able to shift
speech discrimination performance by nearly 30% by simply
focusing attention to the task or by giving the task some
type of visual or motivational pay-off. It would appear that
this kind of modification in the intelligibility task could
easily take place during the evaluative process and could
alter intelligibility performance in a manner that would
readily be interpreted as being clinically significant.
Thus, an aging individual could be credited with achieving

excellent performance with some type of amplification device
when, in fact, the credit might well be given to the situation rather than to the device.

Another excellent mechanism designed for use during
the evaluation and fitting process is the Feasibility Scale
for Predicting Hearing Aid Use as described recently by Rupp,
Higgins and Maurer (1977). Their scale utilizes 11 prognos-
tic factors and each factor is provided with a weighting
which is a reflection of the relative overall importance of
that factor. The 11 factors, listed according to relative
importance, are motivation and referral, magnitude of hearing
loss, self assessment of listening difficulties, age, manual
hand-finger dexterity, financial resources, significant other
person to assist individual, verbalization as to fault of
communication difficulties, informal verbalizations during
hearing aid evaluation, and visual ability. Each of these
factors is rated on a 1 to 5 scale.

For each factor a rating of 5 indicates the most
positive performance. Thus, for example, if an individual
appears to have relatively high motivation and initiated the
referral for the hearing aid on their own with only a little
prodding from others, they would be given a score of 4.
Similarly, each factor has relatively easy to follow guidelines that allow for a degree of objectivity in completing
the feasibility scale. One of the more objectively scored
factors would be the one that relates to magnitude of hearing
loss and results of amplification. Recall that factor
received the second highest weighting of all 11 factors. In
fact, this factor actually consists of three separate items
and can be scored only after completion of some type of evaluative process using actual hearing aids. This factor takes
into account the magnitude of threshold shift achieved with
a specific hearing aid by comparing the unaided and the aided
speech thresholds. The factor then also includes the actual
speech intelligibility performance on a discrimination task
presented in quiet and a discrimination task presented with
competition at a signal to noise ratio of zero dB.

The factors of "financial resources" and "significant
others" require special consideration. All too often we have
heard audiologists, physicians, hearing aid dealers or others
associated with the delivery of service to the aging individual indicate that financial resources should not be a consideration when determining what is needed for, and what would
be beneficial to, the care of the aging individual. While
these statements may be true in theory, they leave a great
deal to be desired in actual practice. Botwinick (1973) has
pointed out that aging individuals tend to be very cautious,

particularly with financial matters. Testimony before the
Senate Subcommittee on Consumer Interests of the Elderly of
the Special Committee on Aging, Hearing Aids and the Older
American (1973) indicated that there is an estimated six
million Americans over the age of 65 who have enough hearing
loss to be considered candidates for hearing aids and yet
only 21% of this total group actually owns hearing aids.
When we consider the fact that single hearing aids presently
cost between $300 and $550, and binaural hearing aids frequently cost at least twice that much, it is not surprising
that many aging individuals shy away from hearing aid use
even when they recognize the need for such use. We dare not
ignore the financial condition of the aging individual or the
aging couple. Real pressure from any of us for the acquisition of a hearing aid can cause significant internal tensions
and problems. The recipient of the instrument feels pressured into constant and continuous hearing aid use, even when
it might not truly be appropriate, because of the high expenditure of money. The recipient of the hearing aid is frequently very hesitant to report hearing aid malfunctions or
difficulties because of the fear that these may result in
still further expenditures of money. The recipient of the
hearing aid frequently is very hesitant to speak out about
any aspect of the hearing aid that might be unfavorable or
unpleasant because it might look as though they were not getting full benefit from this very expensive prosthetic device.
The family or spouse, on the other hand, tend to feel that
they have been pressured into a large expenditure of money by
being made to feel that their stinginess would greatly impair
the hearing impaired individual's potential for a successful
and happy life. Thus, the hearing aid is actually purchased,
but both the recipient and the family or spouse can be un-
happy or uneasy about the situation that has been created. I
would strongly urge, when dealing with the aging population,
that serious consideration be given to financial resources
before strong recommendations are made for the purchase of an
amplification system.
     The final characteristic on the feasibility scale
deals with the existence of a significant other person. With
the aging individual this is particularly important. Communication does not take place in a vacuum but involves both the
hearing aid user and other speakers, and often, with this
population one primary or significant other individual. Particularly when there are additional problems with manual
dexterity, visual ability, or memory, the significant other
person is of primary importance in determining potential
success. This is the individual who can assist with the

actual physical use of the instrument and who can provide
sympathetic understanding or real help when difficult listening situations make specific listening success difficult or
nearly impossible. Particularly, with the independent aging
individual the significant other person can provide a greater
degree of satisfaction and a higher likelihood of appropriate
hearing aid use than that achieved by the hearing aid user
functioning by themselves.

The next major category of potential hearing aid
users among the aging population are those that are classified as semi-independent. These are individuals who may be
relatively independent in most aspects of life but who are
living with family or friends who play a large part in dic-
tating the life-style of the individual. Frequently, individuals in this category are persons who are physically, mentally, and emotionally independent but who have a real or
imagined financial dependence that causes them to select and
continue with this living mode. Oftentimes, typical evaluative procedures, using relatively standard test materials,
are appropriate for this population. It is critical,
however, for those persons who are controlling the older
individual's life-style to be involved with the complete
evaluation and fitting procedure. All too often, the aging
semi-independent individual, even though highly motivated
and possessing great need, will outrightly reject any consideration of amplification if they feel a negative attitude on
the part of the person or persons controlling their life-
style. The aging individual feels a real need to conduct
themselves in a manner acceptable to the expectations or
beliefs of the person controlling their life-style. If we
can generate a positive and encouraging attitude on the part
of the individual controlling the life-style, we can most
often achieve a positive and encouraging attitude on the part
of the potential hearing aid user. In this instance, the
significant other person would undoubtedly be the friend or
a family member responsible for the living situation.
Indeed, the complete feasibility scale is highly appropriate
for use with the semi-independent individual and is very
valuable in assisting with predictive statements regarding
potential hearing aid use.

The last major category includes the dependent living
older individual. While people within this category possess
a broad continuum of abilities and disabilities, we are generally referring here to those who are found in a nursing
home situation. Oftentimes, these individuals have restric-
ted mobility and, as a result, little or no motivation toward
amplification or communicative improvement. In fact, Gaitz

and Warshaw (1964) and Alpiner (1973) have pointed out a real reticence on the part of nursing home residents to obtain amplification or communicative help even when it can be done at no cost. For many of these individuals, a recommendation for hearing aid use must be made, not necessarily on the basis of need, but on the basis of potential for use and potential for success. Very often, the evaluation must be carried out in the nursing home rather than in an audiology facility. The evaluation must be done with relatively short test intervals and with test material that will be appropriate and have some meaning to the recipient.

In those instances where subject response is not possible due to physical, mental or emotional factors, the benefit of the hearing aid must be determined on the basis of observational data. We must determine whether the individual is capable of responding to voices and environmental sounds, whether the individual can show an awareness to the presence of speech, whether visual contact is altered as a result of hearing aid use, whether there is any reaction (either positive or negative) to loud sound or whether the individual tends to show any overt aggressions toward the hearing aid. While observational data may appear to be somewhat subjective, it should not be surprising that this type of data is frequently very consistent and frequently very meaningful. Even though a significant hearing loss may be known to exist, the potential for any kind of successful hearing aid use is very very limited when observational responses cannot verify a meaningful sound input.

With the dependent living group, it is also essential to ascertain whether or not staff individuals exist who are at least minimally proficient in hearing aid use. If a staff is not interested in hearing aid use, is not willing to learn about the intricacies and nuances of hearing aid use, does not believe that hearing aids would be beneficial with this population, then the potential for any kind of successful use will be very limited. Frequently, the bulk of a total evaluation with dependent living individuals may be spent in trying to teach staff members how to deal with hearing aids and how to ensure that the hearing aid user is actually getting meaningful hearing aid processed sound. Without the knowledgeable support of the nursing facility staff, any kind of successful hearing aid use is almost doomed before it begins.

Two additional conditions, not necessarily related to the process of evaluation and fitting of amplification, should be mentioned in order to be able to present a comprehensive appraisal of potential for success to the aging

individual. Almost everyone associated with the total hearing health scheme has at one time or another reflected upon
the problem of vanity as it effects the potential for hearing
aid use among the aging population. We have considered the
problem created by human vanity, but it is most often felt
that, if we talk logically and convincingly, we could finally
get the aging individual to forget their appearance and think
about their hearing. While our motives may have been admir-
able, our approach to the situation may have been well wide
√ of the mark. While we do not possess strong data that apply
specifically to the aging population, we can borrow from an
intriguing study reported recently by Blood, Blood and
Danhauer (1977) and we can generalize from their data in
terms of its application to the aging population. These
authors simply photographed twelve normal hearing teenagers.
Two pictures were taken of each teenager, one with a hearing
aid on and one without a hearing aid. They also recorded a
one minute speech sample from each teenager. The photographs, along with the speech samples, were presented to 50
college students in such a fashion that each college aged
judge viewed photographs of each teenager either with or
without the hearing aid. No judge viewed both photographs of
the same teenager under both conditions. At the same time
the photograph was being viewed the college aged judge heard
the one minute speech sample. It should be remembered that
the same speech sample was used whether the judge viewed the
photograph of the teenager with the hearing aid on or without
the hearing aid.

Each judge viewed the photograph, heard the speech
sample, and then ranked the teenager on a twenty (20) part
semantic differential scale utilizing adjective pairs. Five
adjective pairs dealing with *intelligence* ranged from extremes such as "intelligent to stupid" or "educated to unedu-
cated". There were also ranking factors relating to
individual *achievement* which ranged from "high achiever to
low achiever" or "successful to unsuccessful". Adjective
pairs that pertained to *personality* ranged from "active to
passive" or "friendly to unfriendly". Under the *appearance*
hearing they were ranked from extremes such as "attractive to
unattractive" or "good looking to plain". Recall that these
were the same children being shown once wearing a hearing aid
and once not wearing a hearing aid.

Remarkably, of the twenty total adjective pairs that
related to intelligence, achievement, personality and appearance, the photographs of the teenagers wearing hearing aids
were ranked significantly poorer for 19 of the 20 factors.
The only factor in which there was not a significant

difference between the hearing aid wearers and the non-hearing aid wearers was the personality factor that ranged from kind to cruel. We should at least take some small pride in the fact that college age judges did not consider teenagers wearing hearing aids as being more cruel than their normal counterparts.

We were particularly intrigued by this rather shocking set of data. We have been involved in attitudinal investigations regarding the aging hearing aid user. Unfortunately, we do not yet have sufficient data to report at this point. However, in order to obtain informal data I recently attended a meeting with several young to middle-aged businessmen. During the course of the proceedings I posed this situation. I indicated to them that they walked into a room and found four older individuals. One of the four older individuals was wearing a hearing aid. I then requested that each person present come up with a single word or a single phrase that would most accurately describe the aging individual who was wearing the hearing aid. The terms provided by this group of businessmen included such items as "senile, in need of help, unable to care for self, probably not with it, way over the hill" and "to be avoided". Depressingly, every single statement regarding the aging hearing aid user was made in a negative or derogatory vein and not one single statement had anything to do with the fact that the individual was hard of hearing or may have had difficulty with their hearing. The general impression to be gained from these statements from young and middle-aged businessmen was that the aging hearing aid user had taken leave of their faculties, if indeed they ever had faculties to begin with. Unfortunately, I do not think that this informal sample is very far from the real life situation. It simply but clearly points out the fact that we must keep these attitudes continually in mind and we must work constantly with family members, friends or care staff who come in daily or occasional contact with the aging hearing aid user to orient them to the real meaning of hearing aid use.

One final factor should be dealt with. We have discussed in general, factors or conditions that should be a part of our considerations during the evaluation and fitting process. Once the aging individual owns a hearing aid, however, they must be prepared to keep it in proper operating condition. This will mean that they have to initiate repair services when the instrument malfunctions and, with the aging population, there appears to be a higher rate of instrument abuse and instrument malfunction. Recently, Warren and Kasten (1976) reported the results of an investigation in

which they evaluated the performance of hearing aids that had
been repaired in manufacturer's repair facilities and in alternative repair facilities. These authors examined only the
appropriateness of gain, saturation sound pressure level and
frequency response and related the condition of these characteristics after repair to those specified by the manufacturer
for that model of aid. They found that, regardless of the
type of repair facility used, 39% of the instruments returned
to the user from the repair facility actually possessed
appropriate characteristics. In fact, almost 10% still
possessed such gross malfunctions that they had to be returned to the repair facility again before they could even be
evaluated. If we simply consider the reticence on the part
of some aging individuals to spend additional money and generalize the cautiousness characteristic of some aging individuals, it is easy to see how an improperly repaired hearing
aid could cause an older individual to give up and cease
hearing aid use rather than complain or argue for additional
service. An example of the kind of problem that could con-
front the aging individual is taken from Kasten and Braunlin
(1970) who reported on a modification to a hearing aid for
which they requested a modification that would provide
approximately 30 dB of gain and 100 dB of saturation. When
the instrument was returned to them it was more powerful than
when originally sent in. The aid was returned to be modified
to deliver 30 dB of gain and 100 dB of output and came back
to them again delivering more power than when they had originally started. Once again the instrument went back to the
manufacturer and was returned. This modification was also
rejected and the instrument went back to the manufacturer and
was returned once more. Once again they were far from the
requested characteristics. The fifth factory modification
actually achieved the desired characteristics.

      This information is not meant to be a condemnation of
repair programs, but simply to illustrate the kind of problems that can develop and could confound successful use by
the aging individual. Consistent and meaningful intervention
and advocacy on behalf of the aging individual will be critical for the maintenance of a properly functioning amplification system and the continuance of hearing aid use.

      In summary, I have tried to get across a few basic
ideas. As we talk about the evaluation, a method of getting
a hearing aid to an aging person, and the fitting, the process of putting it on and keeping it on, we have to realize
that we are dealing with a large group of people that are
exceedingly complex in terms of both their abilities and
their disabilities. We have to realize that with many adults

we have, over a number of years, molded the individual to fit our evaluation procedure. With the aging individual it is necessary for us to mold our evaluation to fit the individual. We have to realize, as was stated earlier and I am sure will be stated again, evaluation and fitting is only the beginning; it is only a start and nothing but a start. The hearing aid user and the significant other person or persons must be involved in the total process from the very beginning. The aging individual, if we take the liberty of talking about them as a single entity, will require continued involvement and advocacy on our part in order to ensure continued hearing aid use.

And finally, and probably more important than anything else, aging individuals can be and should be hearing aid users. We have somehow perpetuated the fiction for years that there is something about these people that makes the use of amplification good with only a small percentage of the total group. A great many, far more than presently exist in this population, can and should be successful hearing aid users and they can achieve that goal only with the help of groups like this.

REFERENCES

1. Alpiner, J. G. The Hearing Aid in Rehabilitation Planning for Adults. *Journal of the Academy of Rehabilitative Audiology, 6,* 55-57, 1973.

2. Blood, G. W., Blood, I. M. and Danhauer, J. L. The Hearing Aid "Effect". *Hearing Instruments, 28, 12,* June, 1977.

3. Botwinick, J. Aging and Behavior. New York; Springer, 1973.

4. Chatfield, W. F. Economic and Sociological Factors Affecting Life Satisfaction of the Aged. *Journal of Gerontology, 32,* 593-599, 1977.

5. Cumming, E. and Henry, W. Growing Old, The Process of Disengagement. New York; Basic Books, 1961.

6. Frankel, A. The Eradication of Poverty in Comtemporary America; Genesis, Treatment and Evaluation. *The Journal of Irreproducable Results, 19, 40,* 1972.

7. Gaitz, C. N. and Warshaw, H. E. Obstacles Encountered
    in Correcting Hearing Loss in the Elderly.
    Geriatrics, 19, 83-86, 1964.

8. Gilbert, J. G. and Levee, R. F. Patterns of Declining
    Memory. *Journal of Gerontology, 26,* 70-75, 1971.

9. Kasten, R. N. and Braunlin, R. Traumatic Hearing Aid
    Usage; A Case Study. Paper presented before the
    convention of the American Speech and Hearing
    Association, 1970.

10. Kasten, R. N. and Thomas, P. Unpublished Research
    Conducted at Wichita State University, 1978.

11. Loether, H. J. Problems of Aging. Encino, California;
    Dickenson, 1975.

12. Minnesota Public Interest Research Group, Hearing Aids
    and The Hearing Aid Industry in Minnesota.
    Minneapolis; MPIRG, 1972.

13. Retired Professional Action Group, Paying Through the
    Ear; A Report on Hearing Health Care Problems.
    Philadelphia; Public Citizen, Inc., 1973.

14. Rupp, R. R., Higgins, J. and Maurer, J. F. A
    Feasibility Scale for Predicting Hearing Aid Use
    (FSPHAU) with Older Individuals. *Journal of the
    Academy of Rehabilitative Audiology, 10,* 81-104,
    1977.

15. United States Senate Hearings. Subcommittee on
    Consumer Interests of the Elderly of the Special
    Committee on Aging, Hearing Aids and the Older
    American, September, 1973.

16. Warren, M. P. and Kasten, R. N. Efficacy of Hearing
    Aid Repairs by Manufacturers and by Alternative
    Repair Facilities. *Journal of the Academy of
    Rehabilitative Audiology, 9,* 38-47, 1976.

Chapter 6

Development of a Tactile Aid
For the Profoundly Hearing Impaired:
Implications for Use
With the Elderly

BRIAN L. SCOTT, PH. D.

INTRODUCTION

In the first part of this paper, I will describe a
tactile aid to speech reception. The aid was developed as a
sensory substitution device, that is, it was designed to be
used only by persons unable to benefit from conventional am-
plication. But we now believe that what we have learned
about tactile speech communication can be applied to a much
broader segment of the hearing-impaired population: people
with severe high-frequency hearing losses. We are proposing
that in some cases of high-frequency hearing loss, vibrotactile stimulation may be more beneficial than amplification in
the sensing of high-frequency signals. To support this contention, we will rely on the successes of the tactile aid
project and on recent physiological data which can explain
why amplification can be a problem with high-frequency hearing loss.

I. The Tactile Aid

The Tactile Aid was developed at the Central Institute for the Deaf. Three versions of the aid were construc-
ted and evaluated before we were convinced that we had an aid
with practical value. The first aid was a simple device with
a low-frequency vibratory channel and a single high-frequency
electrocutaneous channel. The results from this aid are
relevant to the discussion of tactile supplements to conventional hearing aids and will therefore be discussed in the
next section. In this section, we will focus on the second
and third generation aids.

First, I would like to briefly describe our evaluation method which has been dubbed the "tracking" procedure
(DeFilippo and Scott, 1978). It is a means of testing a

83

communication channel with ongoing speech. The test material
is prose and, in this case, consisted of two novels. Basically, the procedure works as follows: The subject (or lipreader) is seated opposite the experimenter (or reader).
Normal hearing subjects are functionally deafened with earplugs and noise and are either in an unaided lipreading condition or an aided lipreading condition. The experimenter
begins a ten-minute "trial" by starting a timer and beginning
to read from the text. The experimenter determines how much
to read at a time and that may vary from as little as a single word to as much as a seven or eight-word sentence. The
subject responds by attempting to repeat verbatim what the
experimenter has read. Errors are corrected exclusively
through verbal means. At the end of the ten-minute interval,
the clock is stopped and the number of words of text read by
the experimenter are counted. The word count does not include corrections or repetitions, therefore the fewer the
errors, and more rapid the communication rate, the higher the
word count. The exact time and words of text covered are
then used to derive the words-per-minute score which you will
see on the ordinate of all our data figures.
         The first aid we are going to discuss is shown sche-
matically in Figure 1. We have called this aid the "hybrid"
aid because of the combination of electrocutaneous stimulation with vibrotactile stimulation for the transduction of
the signal. As can be seen from the schematic, the speech
signal is processed in three channels. The high-frequency
channel consists of a high-pass filter at 8 kHz, followed by
an envelope detector and an electrical pulse generator[1].
Pulses are bipolar and occur at a fixed burst rate (156 per
second). Changes in intensity are coded by varying number of
pulses per burst, which is determined by the amplitude of the
envelope of the high-passed signal. The transducers are bipolar, concentric, silver electrodes. The mid-frequency
channel is also electrical but differs in that the speech
signal is bandpassed at 2.4 kHz and the resultant electrical
pulses are conveyed to two electrodes instead of one. The
low-frequency channel consists of a bandpass filter with a
low cutoff at 250 Hz and high cutoff at 900 Hz. The

---

[1]The electrical pulse generator was developed by Frank
Saunders and is described in Saunders, F. A. (1974), "Electrocutaneous displays", Conference on Vibrotactile Communication, edited by F. A. Geldard (The Psychonomic Society,
Austin, Texas), P. 25.

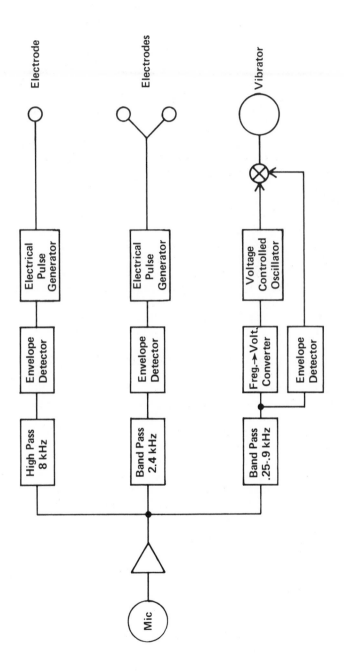

FIG. 1. Block diagram of the tactile aid. This version of the aid utilizes both the electrocutaneous and vibrotactile stimulation as shown.

85

bandpassed signal is sent in parallel through a frequency-to-voltage converter and an envelope detector. The output voltage of the converter is used to drive a voltage controlled oscillator, the output of which is then multiplied by the envelope of the original signal. In essence, the electronics in the low-frequency channel accomplished a frequency transposition of the first formant of vowel sounds. The transposed signal is then delivered to a Suvag vibrator. Figure 2 shows how the transducers are worn.

The electrodes are arranged on the back of the hand. The center electrode carries the high-frequency information and the outside electrodes carry the mid-frequency information. The vibrator on the back of the wrist is the low-frequency channel and conveys the frequencies between 250 and 900 Hz transposed down to between 20 and 200 Hz. The sensation elicited by high frequencies is electrical, punctate, and aperiodic. The sensation from the mid-frequency channel is electrical, diffuse, and aperiodic, the diffuse sensation being a function of both outside electrodes carrying the same information and thus stimulating a much larger area than the single high-frequency electrode. The sensation from the low-frequency channel is vibratory and varies in "roughness" and "smoothness" with changes in first format frequency.

The subjects in the first experiment were the experimenters. Both had had training in lipreading (about 50-60 hours per subject), unaided and aided, although not with the present aid. The training and testing were done with the tracking procedure. The subjects had had approximately three hours experience with the present aid prior to the beginning of this experiment. The experiment consisted of five hours (30 10-minute intervals) lipreading alone followed by five hours of aided lipreading. The first five hours of data will thus establish an unaided lipreading baseline, for two well-trained subjects, with which to compare the second five hours of aided lipreading data. Data are shown in Figure 3.

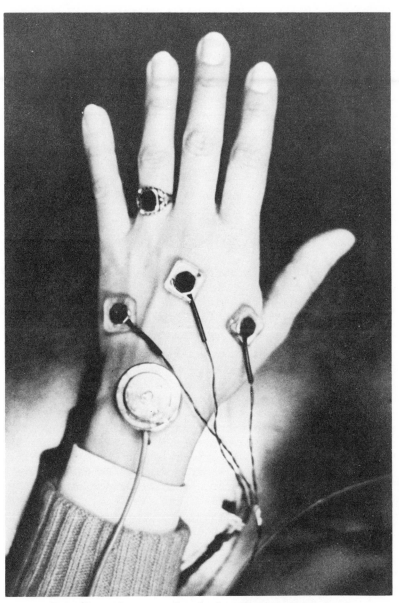

FIG. 2. Photograph of the three electrical and single vibratory transducers as worn on the back of the hand. The center electrode conveys high-frequency information, the electrodes on either side convey mid-frequency information, and the vibrator conveys low-frequency information.

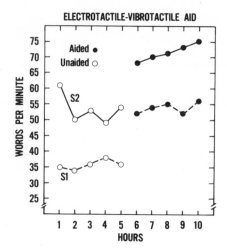

FIG. 3.   Tracking data from two subjects.
The lipreading-alone data (open circles) is
followed by data from subjects lipreading
with the tactile aid (filled circles).

The solid lines are for S2 and the dashed, for S1.
As you can see, changing from unaided lipreading to aided
lipreading has a marked effect on performance. To get a reference for the word-per-minute score, consider performing
the tracking task in a normal hearing mode, that is, without
the plugs and noise. For this team, the tracking rate in the
normal hearing mode is approximately 100 wpm. Thus, in the
last hour of testing, S1 is performing at better than half
of normal rate and S2 at three-fourths of normal rate. We
might also suggest, from these data, that this does not represent asymptotic performance.
        There are two separate aspects to the next experi-
ment: (1) an all-vibratory version of the aid will be described, and (2) the subjects are totally naive lipreaders.
There were two reasons for using naive rather than trained
subjects. First, we wanted to know if using the aid could
help train lipreading. In other words, does one have to be
a sophisticated lipreader in order to appreciate and benefit
from information conveyed tactually, or can this information
actually help the naive observer learn the visual skill of
lipreading? The second reason was to see how much experience
with the aid would be necessary before differences in aided
and unaided scores would appear.

The vibratory aid is shown schematically in Figure 4. The major difference between this aid and the former is that this one is all-vibratory. We decided that there would be some advantages to an all-vibratory system over our hybrid vibratory-electrical system after encountering problems with large threshold shifts for electrical stimulation due to subtle changes in electrode placements. Another reason for going to an all-vibratory display was to avoid anticipated resistance to the use of electrical stimulation with very young subjects. This schematic represents our solution to the problem of conveying the same kind of information we had in our former aid with an all vibrator display. Again, we have three channels with filter characteristics identical to those of the former aid. The difference is that now the energy in the top two filters is used to modulate the amplitude of a noise source rather than to determine the amount of electrical stimulation. The noise source is bandpass-filtered at 250 Hz and infinitely peak-clipped prior to multiplication so that the output will more faithfully follow the envelope of the input signal. The bottom, low-frequency channel is identical to that of the former aid but the output is directed to all transducers. The vibrator carrying the high-frequency information is worn between the vibrators carrying the mid-frequencies. The center vibrator carries the high frequencies and vowels and the outside vibrators convey the mid-frequencies and vowels. To describe the sensation from using this aid, a change from /s/ to /sh/ causes the aperiodic noise sensation to spread from the center, outward. A change from /s/ to a vowel causes both spreading and a change from the aperiodic to a periodic sensation with a concomitant drop in frequency.

The vibrators are secured just below the rib cage by an elastic band. The change in location from the back of the hand was necessitated by the increase in size of the transducers. The loss in sensitivity from going to the torso appears to be more than compensated for in terms of convenience.

There were eight normal hearing subjects in this experiment divided into four teams. The members of a team switched between experimenter (reader) and subject (lipreader). Two teams were in the all-vibratory aid condition, and two in the hybrid aid condition. In a given aid condition, one team lipread alone without the aid, for a total of four hours (24 10-minute trials), then switched to the aided condition. The other team began with the aid, and switched after four hours to lipreading alone. Figure 5 shows the results from the all-vibratory aid.

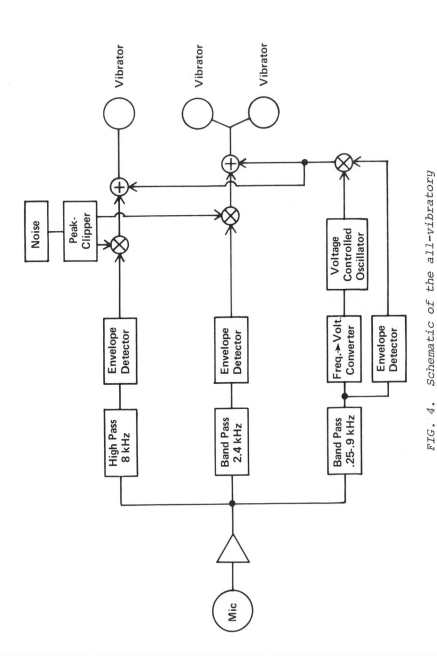

FIG. 4. Schematic of the all-vibratory version of the tactile aid.

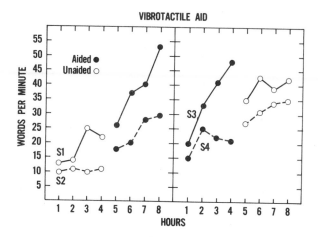

FIG. 5. Results showing the effectiveness of the all-vibratory aid. Panel "a" shows data from subjects who lipread unaided for 4 hours, then lipread with the aid for 4 hours. Panel "b" shows data for subjects that lipread with the aid first, followed by lipreading without the aid.

The left panel shows the data from the team which lipread for four hours and then switched to using the aid. For both subjects, the rate of learning to lipread increased considerably as indicated by the increase in the slope of the learning curves from the unaided to the aided condition. The panel on the right is for the team which used the aid initially and then went to lipreading alone. Subject three showed very rapid learning over the first four hours with the aid, then fell off in performance when the aid was turned off. The fall-off was not, however, what one would expect if there were no carry-over effect of learning to lipread with the aid. In fact, the lipreading-alone performance of S3 would indicate a considerable acceleration of learning to lipread given use of the aid. Our fourth subject did not show the rate of learning in the aided condition that the others did. This was probably due to the fact that this subject found the sensation uncomfortable and complained of some nausea. On the whole, we believe these data indicate that a subject can learn to utilize the aid with very little training (recall that these subjects had never before done any lipreading), and that using the aid can help one to learn how to lipread.

Figure 6 shows the data from the hybrid aid.

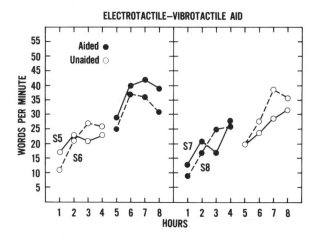

FIG. 6. *Data from hybrid electrocutaneous-vibrotactile aid. Same conditions as in Figure 5.*

Unfortunately, these data are quite ambiguous. There are no large differences in the slopes of the aided versus the unaided learning curves with the possible exception of those of S5. Perhaps the only indication that the aid is really doing anything is the decrement in performance in the right panel after the aid is turned off (see hour 5), but this decrement soon disappears with further experience lipreading alone. We feel there are at least two possible reasons for not finding the same encouraging results found with the all-vibratory aid. The most likely is that it was more difficult to obtain a good, reliable sensation from the electrical channels due to our poor choice of location, that is, the bony back of the hand. The other possibility is that it simply takes longer to learn to integrate the electrical with the vibratory stimulation and therefore more training is necessary than the four hours we allowed our subjects. We do not believe these data to be indicative of the potential of the hybrid electrical-vibratory aid since our well-trained subjects achieved 56% and 75% normal listening rate.

II. A Vibratory Aid for High-Frequency Hearing Loss

In this section we will explore the possibility of using a vibrotactile aid for conveying just the high frequencies of speech. In this application, a tactile aid would compliment a conventional hearing aid by providing a vibrotactile display of sounds like /s/ and /sh/, while the hearing aid provided information about the lower frequencies of speech (the vowels).

In the first part of this section, we will discuss some physiological problems with the use of amplification in cases of extreme presbycusis. In the second part we will discuss the use of a tactile aid as an alternative to amplification for high-frequency hearing loss.

A. The Physiological Basis for a Vibratory Display of High frequencies

1. A physiological Mechanism for the Compensation of Hair Cell Loss

For decades, there have been arguments in the hearing science literature over whether the ear codes the acoustic waveform temporally, spatially or through a combination of the two. Spatial coding, of course, refers to recognizing frequency components of a signal by the location along the basilar membrane of maximum displacement. Temporal coding refers to the analysis of spectral information by rate of neural firing. There now seems to be little doubt that both mechanisms are in play; the only question being the magnitude of the role each plays. Sachs & Young (1978) have provided evidence, using single-unit recording techniques, that place information in the coding of vowel sounds is significant only at lower sound levels, and only for vowels with widely spaced formants. Temporal coding seems to be the more important means of analyzing vowel information in the ear.

Our interest in this seemingly subtle distinction stems from the greater redundancy in temporal coding than spatial coding. _Any_ neuron firing once every ten milliseconds is conveying information about a hundred Hertz stimulus. Only those neurons excited by hair cells lying at a specific location on the basilar membrane can convey spatial information about a one hundred Hertz stimulus. The redundancy of temporal coding provides a "back-up" system for protection against losing the hair cells tuned to lower frequencies. The temporal firing patterns of other neurons will

insure that we can still perceive those frequencies even when
there has been considerable damage in the low-frequency por-
tions of the cochlea.

The redundancy of temporal and spatial coding of low
frequencies provides protection against the loss of spectral
resolution in the low frequencies. The ear also provides a
"back-up" mechanism to protect against extreme losses in sensitivity. In order to illustrate this second "back-up" mechanism and to indicate the possible significance in hearing
problems, I'm going to describe some recent physiological
data collected by Dr. John Markuszka at the Central Institute
for the Deaf. Dr. Markuszka was interested in the discrep-
ency between behavioral data and anatomical damage found in
studies on noise-induced hearing losses in animals (Ward and
Duvall, 1971). In general, behaviorally measured hearing
thresholds are found to be considerably better than would be
predicted from the amount of hair cell damage observed under
microscopic examination. In the Ward and Duvall (1971)
study, two chinchillas were exposed to a band of noise two
octaves wide (710-2800 Hz) at 123 dB SPL for fifteen minutes.
One animal was sacrificed after seven days with a 20 dB behaviorally-determined threshold shift and the other after
fourteen days with no remaining threshold shift (indicating
total recovery). Anatomical evaluations of the cochleas revealed a dramatic loss of outer hair cells. The authors concluded that: "Apparently, normal IHC's (inner hair cells)
are sufficient for a normal pure tone threshold".

Markuszka (in preparation) used single unit record-
ings to study the effects of noise on the cochleas of chinchillas. In this technique, a micro-electrode is used to
record the responses of single neural fibers in the eighth
nerve after exposure to noise. Using this technique, threshold shifts 35-45 dB greater than those found behaviorally
(Carder and Miller, 1972) were observed. It is Markuszka's
explanation of why the discrepancy between single-unit and
behavioral data exists that is of importance to us.

In Figure 7, we can see good agreement between the
behavioral audiogram, shown as the solid line along the
bottom of the figure, (Miller and Carder, 1972), and the
single-unit data from normal chinchillas (Markuszka, in
preparation).

In Figure 8, we see the effects on single-units of
an eight hour exposure of an octave band of noise centered
at 500 Hz at 95 dB SPL.

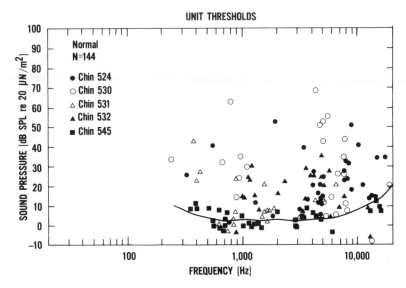

FIG. 7. Single-unit thresholds as recorded
from five normal chinchillas. Solid line is
the behaviorally-determined normal thresholds
of chinchillas as measured by Carder and
Miller (1972).

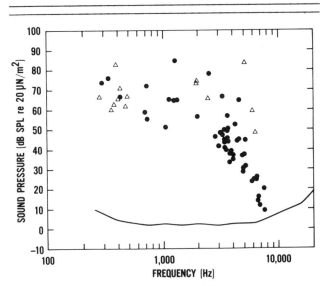

FIG. 8. Single-unit thresholds after an
eight-hour exposure to an octave band of
noise centered at 500 Hz.

The solid line is the normal threshold determined by Carder
and Miller (1972) and is presented as a reference. The elevation in threshold shown here around the center frequency of
the noise is 60-70 dB. This elevation is 35-45 dB greater
than that shown by Carder and Miller behaviorally with an
identical noise exposure. In order to explain this discrepancy, we must look at the tuning curves of the neurons. In
Figure 9, we see tuning curves of several neurons from normal
animals.

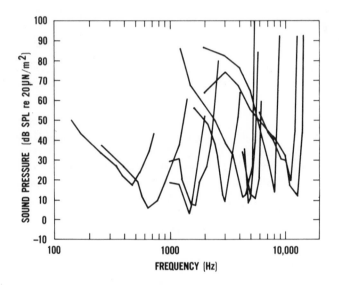

FIG. 9. Tuning curves taken from normal chinchillas. Note the typical sharp tuning of the
high-frequency units and broad tuning of the
low-frequency units. Note also the typical
low-frequency "tails" of the tuning curves.

Note the typical sharp tuning of high-frequency units and
broad tuning of low frequency units. In Figure 10, we see
the tuning curves of several units from the 8-hour noise
exposed animals.

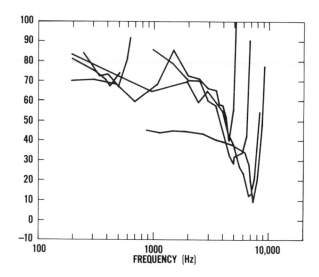

FIG. 10. *Tuning curves of units from chin-chillas exposed to eight hours of an octave band of noise centered at 500 Hz. Note the normal shapes of the tuning curves of high-frequency units and the distorted shapes of the tuning curves of the low-frequency units. The "tails" of the tuning curves tend to mask the threshold shifts of the low-frequency units.*

In the region of the exposure (500 Hz), the tuning curves are distorted as well as elevated. But note the normal appearance of the high-frequency units, particularly the one centered at about 7500 Hz. This unit shows the typical steep slope on the high-frequency side of the tuning curve and the long, broadly-tuned "tail" on the low-frequency side. It is the presence of this "tail" that explains the descrepency between the single-unit thresholds and the behavioral thresholds. The unit tuned to a frequency of 7500 Hz will fire to a 1000 Hz tone just 35 dB above its threshold at 7500 Hz. Markuszka hypothesized that the smaller behaviorally determined threshold shifts are a function of exciting normal high-frequency neurons before reaching the thresholds of the damaged neurons in the actual region of noise exposure. Thus,

it is the broadly-tuned low-frequency tails of neural tuning
curves that provides the mechanism for minimizing threshold
shifts caused by acoustic trauma.

This experiment provides a glimpse into the elegant
nature of how the auditory system provides "back-up" mechanisms to minimize damage. Even the total destruction of hair
cells in a specific frequency region can be compensated for.
The tails of the tuning curves of higher frequency neurons
will insure a limited threshold shift and the ability to
phase-lock will insure frequency discrimination. The effectiveness of this system depends however, on the presence of
healthy neurons in the higher frequency regions. The tuning
curves are asymmetrical with tails only on the low-frequency
side. Thus, units with center-frequencies lower than the
site of damage can probably do little in compensating for the
missing hair cells.

2.   Implications for Compensatory Amplification

I would now like to relate the hypothesized compensation mechanism discussed above to the use of amplification in
hearing disorders. The major assumption is that the compensation mechanism theory is accurate, that is, that high-
frequency fibers can compensate for the loss of lower-fre-
quency hair cells by virtue of their broad, low-frequency
tuning and phase-locking properties. Given this assumption,
amplification should be beneficial to anyone with some high-
frequency hearing, regardless of their low-frequency hearing
loss. This residual hearing may be well above the eight
thousand Hertz limit of most audiometers and still be of tremendous benefit in speech reception. Amplifying the speech-
relevant frequencies into the tails of the tuning curves of
the remaining high-frequency fibers will allow the phase-
locking properties of those fibers to extract important low-
frequency information about the speech signal. The obvious
suggestion here is to extend the range of frequencies tested
in audiometric evaluations to well above 8 kHz, particularly
in the case of an individual showing a severe-to-profound
loss below 8 kHz.

But what of the profound high-frequency hearing loss
with relatively normal low-frequency hearing? In this case,
amplification may be contra-indicated given the validity of
the theory. The tails of the tuning curves all extend toward the low-frequencies. The high-frequency side of the
tuning curve is quite steep, indicating the difficulty of
firing the unit with a signal higher in frequency. Thus,
amplifying a high-frequency signal until it is picked up by

a low-frequency unit probably results in considerable distortion of the signal. In fact, it may only be the distortion which is heard. But this isn't necessarily bad. Even if certain speech sounds (such as /s/) are perceived as distortions, they are still perceived. But there must be a limit to this logic. The more severe the high-frequency hearing loss, the more distortion one must put up with in order to squeeze all the relevant speech elements into the remaining hearing. It is for those persons suffering from a severe high-frequency hearing loss that we are proposing the use of a tactile supplement to the conventional hearing aid.

B. Evidence for the Efficacy of a Single-Channel Aid

The first generation of the tactile aid was a simple two-channel device pairing the Suvag vibrator with a single electrocutaneous channel. In evaluating this aid, we compared lipreading alone with lipreading with just the vibrator and with the vibrator plus the high-frequency channel. The vibrator condition without the high-frequency channel approximates the condition of the profoundly deaf child using a hearing aid (Erber, 1974). A comparison of the conditions in our study should provide a rough estimate of what a high-frequency channel can add to speech reception performance.

The low-frequency vibratory channel consisted of an amplifier, a low pass filter at 1000 Hz (24 dB per octave), and the Suvag vibrator. The high-frequency electrotactile channel consisted of a high pass at 4000 Hz, an electrical pulse generator (as used with the hybrid aid described above), and a silver, bipolar electrode. Both transducers are shown in Figure 11. The electrode was worn on the back of the hand between the thumb and forefinger. The Suvag was worn on the palm opposite the electrode.

The subjects were the experimenters, two normal hearing adults functionally deafened with earplugs and noise during the experiment. The experimental procedure was the "tracking" procedure described above. Subjects had had 10-13 hours experience with the aid prior to the collection of these data. In this experiment, the subjects changed conditions after each 10 minute interval so that data from all three conditions were collected in parallel. The data are shown in Figure 12.

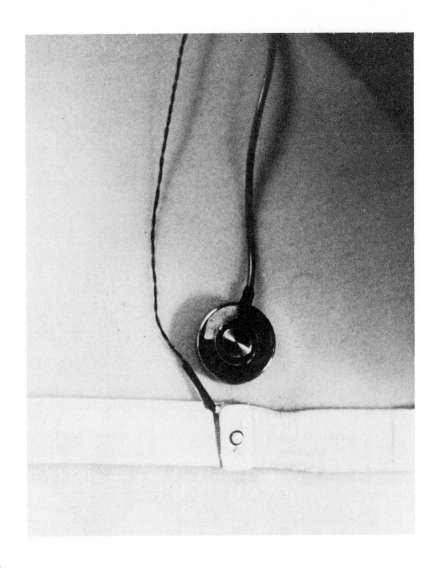

FIG. 11. *Single electrode and vibrator used as transducers for the first tactile aid. Electrode conveyed high-frequency information and the vibrator conveyed the amplitude envelope of the speech signal.*

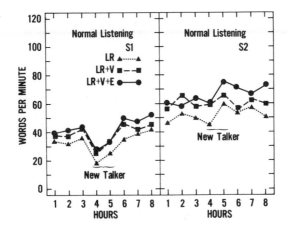

FIG. 12. Tracking data showing lipreading-
alone performance (diamonds), lipreading
with a single vibrator (squares), and lipreading with the vibrator and electrical
channel (circles).

The dotted line represents the rate of unaided lipreading, the dashed line is the rate of lipreading with just
the vibrator and the solid line is the rate of lipreading
with both vibrator and electrical channels. During hours 4
and 5, the speaker was changed to see what the effect would
be on lipreading performance. The change had the same effect
on all three conditions.

The addition of the vibrator elevated lipreading performance by 20% for subject 1 (S1) and 16% for subject 2 (S2)
relative to lipreading-alone performance. This improvement
is somewhat better than the 7% to 11% improvement that

Erber (1972) found with deaf children using hearing aids,
relative to their lipreading-alone performance.

The statistic we are specifically concerned with here
is the 7% and 9% (S1 and S2 respectively) improvement found
with the addition of the high-frequency channel. Although
the improvement is somewhat marginal, it does indicate a potential for a high-frequency vibratory supplement to the
hearing aid.

C. A Design for a Tactile Supplement to the Hearing Aid

We are using the coding principles devised for the
second and third generation aids in designing the tactile
supplement to the hearing aid. With these aids, high and
mid-frequency signals can be discriminated along a punctate/
diffuse dimension. Designing this dimension into the hearing
aid supplement would allow the user to discriminate sounds
such as /s/ and /sh/. This should provide a greater increment in speech reception performance than the 7%-9% improvement we found with the single high-frequency channel.

The proposed unit is shown in Figure 13.

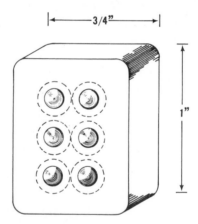

FIG. 13. Proposed vibratory transducer for
high-frequency hearing loss. The six circles
are punctate vibrators activated by high-
frequency signals (8 kHz and above). Mid-
frequency signals (2.4 kHz) activate entire
faceplate of the vibrator.

The transducer must be small enough to be concealed behind the ear. The dimensions shown here are roughly those of a Radio Ear B-70 vibrator. The six small circles in the center of the face plate are the punctate vibrators for conveying the high frequencies of speech. An /s/ sound would cause these small points to vibrate aperiodically with a center frequency of about 250-300 Hz. A mid-frequency signal of about 2500 Hz would cause the entire face-plate to vibrate aperiodically at about 250-300 Hz. The differences in the surface areas of the stimulators provide the punctate/diffuse dimension.

This device is obviously in the germinal stage of planning. There are many problems that have not yet been taken into account. It does, however, represent an alternative approach to the problem of aural rehabilitation for the elderly.

REFERENCES

1. Carder, H. M. and Miller, J. D., "Temporary threshold shifts from prolonged exposure to noise", *J. Speech Hear. Res.*, *15*, 603-623, 1972.

2. DeFilippo, C. L. and Scott, B. L., "A method for training and evaluating the reception of ongoing speech", *J. Acoust. Soc. Am.*, *63*, 1186-1192, 1978.

3. Erber, N. P., "Speech-envelope cues as an acoustic aid to lipreading for profoundly deaf children", *J. Acoust. Soc. Am.*, *51*, 1224-1227, 1972.

4. Erber, N. P., "Visual perception of speech by deaf children: Recent developments and continuing needs", *J. Speech Hear. Dis.*, *39*, 178-185, 1974.

5. Markuszka, J., "The growth of temporary threshold shift in the chinchilla as evidenced in the activity of cochlear neurons", (in preparation).

6. Sachs, M. B. and Young, E. D., "Patterns of auditory nerve fiber responses to steady-state vowels", *J. Acoust. Soc. Am.*, *63*, S76, 1978.

7. Ward, W. D. and Duvall, A. J., "Behavioral and ultrastructural correlates of acoustic trauma", *Ann. Otol.*, *80*, 881-895, 1971.

DISCUSSION

Cooper: Richard Stream, you made some points to me
which I think are very germane to some of the issues that
Roger Kasten and Harriet Kaplan brought up. I would like
you to make your comments at this time.

Stream: First, I would like to thank the speakers
today for their informative and stimulating presentations.
The information presented today has prompted me to make a
comment which concerns the use of students in therapy. Although the underlying assumption is that we are in a helping
profession, I do not believe we should be providing our services free of charge. I make this statement because I am an
advocate for audiologists paying their own way. When we provide hearing therapy services to people at no charge through
training programs we establish an artificial situation in
that we presume these services will be purchased later. However, when the student goes into practice he finds his service is not marketable. The result is that we have professionals to provide a service for which few are willing to
pay. Until we can provide a service that people feel is
worth paying for, we are not going to be able to market it.

Cooper: Before we get on, I think this is an important enough issue that I would like either Harriet Kaplan or
Roger Kasten, or both of them, to respond. The issue is,
basically, should universities pass out free services and, in
effect, undercut their graduates as soon as they walk out the
door with a degree.

Kaplan: I think it is unfortunate that this kind of
therapy is not marketable. I think it is not marketable
because we are dealing with a population that cannot afford
it, regardless of whether they value it or not, and there are
no third party payments at this point that will cover the
cost of this therapy. I think perhaps our emphasis ought to
go toward stimulating third party payments to cover aural
rehabilitation services rather than cutting it off completely. As far as training students, I would not want to stop
training students in this area for a number of reasons.
First of all this ability may become marketable, and secondly, this kind of therapy ought to go hand in hand with
hearing aid evaluation work which does go on in private practice. I do know of some situations where younger adults are
willing to pay for package deals whereby it is one sum to

cover basic evaluation, hearing aid evaluation, and an aural
rehabilitation package. So, I agree with you. There is a
problem, a serious problem, but I do not think the answer is
to eliminate the service.

Kasten: I think there is one other point, Rich
(Stream), that does not necessarily pertain to the service.
As I look at what we are doing I find that one of the big
problems is the fact that we tend to be living in an instant
environment. If we want something to eat, we go to a place
that provides us with instant food. If we want to be enter-
tained, we go someplace that provides us with instant enter-
tainment. If we want to be fixed because there is something
wrong, we go find somebody who can provide an instant fix
and we are okay. If we cannot hear, we get a hearing aid
because that is instant help. Now we are saying, "but we
have something else that is even better than that, except it
takes time", and people do not seem to want to spend time.
They want whatever they are getting now. If we go back 25
years, maybe 30 years, and talk to some of the people who
were involved with the old leagues for the hard of hearing
or community centers for the hearing impaired, we find that
they really taught rehabilitation courses. They called them
by a variety of names but they had rehabilitation courses for
the hearing impaired that went afternoon and night, every day
of the week, and they had people showing up because people
then accepted the fact that this was the one way they could
be helped. In order to receive the help, they had to invest
something into it themselves, and one of the investments was
time. And very frankly, I think much of what we are trying
to say right now, much of what people have been saying for
the past six or seven or eight years is, "Hey, let us wake up
to what we are doing. Let us acknowledge the fact that this
is something that cannot be fixed in an instant." Until
people beging to relearn, until we reinvent the wheel, we are
going to have to drag along. Until we reteach, we are stuck
with having to demonstrate that it can be done and one of the
few ways that we can afford to demonstrate is by using
students.

Stream: I have a question for Dr. Scott. I would
be interested to know if sensitivity to vibration is decreased with the aging of the skin to the extent that the
sort of device you have discussed becomes less effective? I
would also like to comment that I am very interested in seeing if we can get the hearing impaired population, audiologists and engineers to sit down together and work out some

of these ideas for devising better communication instruments. My experience suggests that audiologists sometimes
think the hearing impaired need one thing, but we do not
listen to what they believe they need and neither do the engineers. Perhaps a brainstorming session among these groups
could resolve some of these disparities.

Scott: Your point about aging and skin sensitivity
is very well taken. One nice thing about the skin is that
there is a whole lot of it and if you have specific areas of
insensitivity then that presents a problem. Another aspect,
we are not even approaching the limitations of the skin in
terms of the frequencies that we are using. Now for example, a periodic signal is being coded at roughly 250 Hz. In
an aging person they do not have skin sensitivity at 250 Hz.
We can lower it to 100 Hz or 75 Hz to where they do. We end
up with a slight sacrifice in terms of how well we can
define very rapid changes on the skin, but we can still provide that person with some information. For example, it
might become more difficult to know the difference between
/sa/ and /ta/. It is very simple to perceive when we are
dealing with a 250 Hz signal but the point here is that the
skin can detect vibrations up to about 1000 Hz quite
readily. The skin can discriminate frequencies up to
approximately 250 Hz before the frequencies appear to run
together. We have a lot of margin in terms of our coding
technique.

Your point of drawing people together from different
disciplines, is very well taken. It is very necessary. I
was fortunate enough to be invited to a meeting of the
Rehabilitation Service Administration last May in San
Francisco and there were psychologists, engineers, members
of the deaf community, and as a matter of fact, a representative of Ma Bell. It was incredible, I think, to all of
us, to see how little we knew about everyone else's concerns. Some of the incredible anecdotes that came out, particularly from the from the deaf members of the community,
were astounding. I will not go into those, but I think the
most dramatic example to me was the distance between the
engineers and the people who were actually going to be using
those devices. I have certainly felt a whole lot of that
here today.

Margaret Pete: Could the size of the vibrator ultimately come down to the size of the transcutaneous nerve
stimulator, a TNS unit? This is a device developed which
sends a vibratory signal to the skin to short circuit pain.
They are basically used in orthopedic and spinal cord
injuries. There are two electrode or four electrode monitor

channel units and they are a little larger than a cigarette package and a little bit thinner. Some of the materials that they have may be usable for what you are working for.

Have you looked at high frequency hearing aids for people who have some hearing at 2000 Hz but little or nothing above? This is the population we see that wants ability to know someone is talking. They need some help with the high frequency placed consonants and are not getting it.

Scott: These are precisely the people that we are aiming at; that we would like to see. For that group it might be very good to have just a single channel rather than the dual channel that I outlined here. It might provide them with a lot of benefits.

Chapter 7

The Use of Situational Cues in
Visual Communication

DEAN C. GARSTECKI, PH. D.

I would like to discuss visual communication evaluation and training material which is currently being developed
for use in audiologic rehabilitation of the elderly adult.
Although this material is not yet in its final form, some
preliminary findings with prototype materials have been found
to have important implications for rehabilitation.

Rather than using traditional measures of speechreading ability which have limited prescriptive value, we attempted to isolate and control variables inherent in everyday
communication. Our intent was to identify those variables
which might contribute to and/or interfere with a person's
ability to understand everyday conversation. Information
gleaned from this sample could then be used to develop the
elderly adult's ability to use compensatory cues under everyday communication conditions.

Variables explored included the following:

a) visible speech cues. This refers to use of articulatory posturing and facial expression cues to
understand spoken messages which are masked by competing auditory signals, i.e., conversation in a
noisy subway train.

b) audible speech cues. This refers to use of
audition-only to understand spoken messages which
are not accompanied by cues to articulatory posturing
or facial expression, i.e., speaking to someone from
another room, poor articulator mobility on the part
of the speaker, limited visual acuity or lack of
visible speech cue perception on the part of the
listener, etc.

c) combined visible and audible speech cues. This
refers to use of combined input modalities to

understand spoken messages such as under normal,
everyday communication conditions.

d) environmental cues. This refers to use of
non-verbal auditory and visual situational cues
to spoken message perception, i.e., cafeteria noise
and/or a dining room scene accompanying a conversation relating to restaurant management.

e) linguistic cues. This refers to use of the flow
of English language syntax to predict words in sentences which might be masked by a competing auditory
signal and/or misperceived due to hearing impairment.

The target population for whom this approach is intended comprises the largest category of patients served by the
Northwestern University audiologic rehabilitation program at
this time. These are elderly adults who have either had
normal hearing most of their lives and now are handicapped
due to acquired auditory dysfunction or those who have a
long-standing history of hearing impairment and now, as an
adult, are experiencing communication problems. To distinguish our program from other services available to the hearing handicapped elderly through North Shore suburb Senior
Citizens Centers and the Chicago Hearing Society, we use a
continuing education program format and refer to the program
as a "Hearing Health Workshop". Through the workshop our
Hearing Clinics provide comprehensive evaluative, educational
and counseling service to each individual participant.
        Our interest in analysis of factors which influence
visual communication stems from the frustration and limited
utility of applying traditional lipreading evaluation and
training procedures in audiologic rehabilitation. In our
experience, the elderly adult who is self-referred or highly
motivated toward rehabilitative service most often requests
lipreading lessons. Most assume that, with training, they
will be able to lipread a football coach's instructions to
his team or watch the 5 o'clock news on television with the
sound turned off! Their ultimate wish is to be able to lipread with enough facility to obviate the need for a hearing
aid. If they seek the services of a traditionally trained
audiologist, they may find that rehabilitation service consists largely of hearing aid evaluation and orientation and
counseling. To acquire the lipreading lessons he desires,
the elderly adult may be referred to or otherwise find lessons provided by a speech-language pathologist or "trained"

layman (ASHA, 1977). So ultimately the hearing handicapped adult often acquires the lipreading lessons he originally desired.

The lipreading lesson scene is typified by a row of hearing-aided, eyeglassed, silver-haired senior citizens seated around a table dutifully guessing at every syllable rolling off the instructor's sub-audible lips. Beyond satisfying what they perceive as an important hearing-health-care need, they are generally motivated by the opportunity to socialize with age peers in an "academic" event or by the challenge of second-guessing the instructor in activities resembling the clue-searching suspense of a Columbo mystery. The major focus is seen as striving for "success in class". Improvement in interpersonal interaction ability takes on secondary importance. The underlying theme becomes one of being a good student and studying or intellectualizing your lipreading lesson material rather than learning to apply the principles of effective communication.

The problems inherent in this approach toward visual communication training are well recognized and have been documented by a number of investigators over the past 30 years. In an effort to provide a meaningful and practical inter-phasing of lesson activity and everyday communication experience, several investigators have incorporated "slice-of-life" material into the rehabilitation program framework. Two of the earliest proponents of this approach were Morkovin and Moore (1944). Their Life Situation films depicted verbal interaction among several people on a topic related to the scene, i.e., the grocery store. The films were developed for use as training materials. Utley (1946) incorporated a "story" subtest in her battery of lipreading tests to afford the lipreader the opportunity to gain cues to message perception through linguistic context. Nielsen (1970) used a short film of two people engaged in in-audible conversation while seated at a breakfast table. The film was used to assess visual communication using situational cues and information anticipated from the logical sequence of events. Finally, a similar technique was employed by Fleming (1972). She developed the "Restaurant Test" which was designed to assess the ability to use the logic and sequence of an everyday event, along with visual speech cues and speaker mannerisms, to decode an in-audible pseudo-dialogue.

Although these investigators and others (Jeffers and Barley, 1971) have logically assumed that situational cues facilitate visual message perception, when various types of cues are incorporated into a speech-reading task, it is difficult to know what is being measured and the prescriptive value of the results. One general assumption is that a situational cue provides a referent which may be less ambiguous and less fleeting than an articulatory posturing. If, in fact, situational cues facilitate visual speech perception and the ability of an adult to use these cues can be measured, they could be incorporated into a program to improve visual communication among the hearing impaired elderly who generally require greater redundancy of information and more time to process everyday communication.

To explore the role of situational cues in visual speech perception by the elderly, a series of studies have been conducted over the past few years.

SURVEY

In the earliest stages of our research, we solicited feedback from twenty elderly adults enrolled in an audiologic rehabilitation program in regard to the benefit they felt they derived from various activities. Each person had been receiving some instruction in speechreading for at least four months and one person was approaching his fifth year of participation in the program! In surveying this group, the consensus was that correct perception of a central theme or topic increased the likelihood of being able to understand a spoken message. Each felt that communication ability improved as the ability to watch for and recall familiar information increased.

Influence of Situational Cues on Speechreading Unrelated
  Sentences

To study the influence of situational cues on speechreading, a list of CID Everyday Speech Sentences (Davis and Silverman, 1968) was prepared for presentation by a female adult talker. Sentence presentation was video tape recorded in the video-mode only. Simultaneously, a videotape camera was used to record photographic slides of everyday scenes. A special effects generator was used to combine the video images from each camera on a split viewing screen. Auditory situational cues were dubbed onto the videotape after video recording.

In the first study, sentence perception was studied under three cue conditions. These included visual and auditory cues unrelated to the main idea of a sentence and sentences presented without either visual or auditory cues (Garstecki, 1976). Under the related cue condition, a sentence such as "Do you like to fly at night?" was presented in

the context of an airport scene with a jet noise in the background. The same sentence might be presented in the context
of a dog show with a siren in the background for the unrelated cue condition. When no cues were provided, each sentence
was presented opposite a blank screen. Sentences were presented to 24 subjects ranging in age from 61 to 87 years
($\bar{X}$ = 73 years). The results demonstrated significantly improved performance under the related cue condition as compared to the unrelated and absent cue conditions. There was
no significant difference between performance under unrelated
and absent cue conditions. Under the related cue condition,
an average of 38% of the sentences were correctly perceived
(SD = 12.7; range = 15-55%). Whereas only 10% were perceived under the absent cue condition (SD = 6.6; range =
5-25%) and 6.3% in the unrelated cue condition (SD = 7.4;
range = 0-20%). As expected situational cues appeared to
activate certain expectations. One conclusion from this
study was that geriatric adults with normal language skills
and the ability to process sensory information, used relevant
cues to facilitate sentence perception.

Although this outcome was expected, several interesting exceptions were noted. Several subjects demonstrated
undifferentiated performance across all cue conditions.
Situational cues neither facilitated nor inhibited sentence
perception for these subjects. Some subjects demonstrated
poorer performance when any type of situation cue was presented regardless of the relationship between cue and sentence topic. A third type of exceptional response was demonstrated by undifferentiated high performance under absent and
related cue conditions. These subjects appeared to be able
to perceive enough information from articulatory posturing
cues to discount the need for situational cue information.
These findings suggest that not all geriatric adults are pre-
disposed to benefit from situational cue information. Some
individuals may require special training to tolerate and/or
use situation cues in visual speech perception or speechreading.

To probe the possibility of an age factor contributing
to overall performance, a group of 21 to 24 year old normal
hearing female university students ($\bar{X}$ = 22 years) was administered the same tape material. The results were similar to
those obtained with the geriatrics, but overall ability was
considerably higher:

    a) Related cue condition - 56.3% correct; SD = 11.4;
and, range = 45-75%.

    b) Absent cue condition - 35% correct; SD = 3.5; and,
range = 30-40%.

c) Unrelated cue condition - 27.5% correct; SD = 8.3;
and, range = 15-35%.

Influence of Situational Cues on Speechreading Related Sentences

In a follow-up study, other parameters of situational
cue influence on speechreading ability were explored. One
question related to the possibility that the type of situational cue, auditory or visual, may influence message perception. A second question was concerned with the fact that
everyday communication usually consists of a logically pro-
gressing dialogue in reference to a particular topic, rather
than a list of unrelated sentences. Finally, the majority of
the hearing impaired population have some functional residual
hearing acuity which affords them the benefit of acoustic
cues to visual speech perception.

We attempted to weigh these factors in a follow-up
study (Wales, Garstecki and Privratsky, 1977). Ten adult
residents of the Indiana Veteran's Home who ranged in age
from 61 to 88 years ($\overline{X}$ = 71.5 years) participated in this
study. Test sentences were generated using similar criteria
as incorporated into the development of CID Everyday Speech
Sentences. In this study, however, each sentence pertained
to an event experienced by each resident on a daily basis.
Visual and auditory situational cues included sights and
sounds commonly encountered in the Veteran's Home.

Videotape preparation included recording the production of each sentence by a female talker in a combined audio-
video mode. Auditory background cues were dubbed onto the
videotape at a +10 dB auditory cue to sentence production
level. The experimental tape contained a combined auditory-
visual presentation of each sentence in the context of visual
and auditory background cues. For half of the sentences, the
situational cues were related. The remaining half were unrelated to each sentence.

Because speech discrimination ability under quiet conditions was generally high among these subjects, the audibility of each sentence was uniformly degraded by mixing sentence playback with white noise and presenting this mixed
signal in a sound field environment at 20 dB SL (re: pure
tone average of the better ear). White noise was regulated
to provide a -6 dB SN ratio. Because the white noise level
was determined in relation to the sentence level and the auditory cues were recorded at a +10 dB SN level, auditory cues
were in effect presented at a low positive (+4 dB) SN ratio.

The results demonstrated that best performance
occurred when related visual cues were provided. The mean
percent correct under related visual cue conditions was 67.4%
(SD = 19.7; range = 36.4 - 90.1%). Under the unrelated visual cue condition, the mean percent correct was 43.6% (SD =
21.5; range = 20-80%). The strong performance under the related visual cue condition was expected in view of the effort
made to insure that the cues were within each subject's
daily experience.

Under auditory cue conditions, no statistically significant difference in performance was noted between related
and unrelated cue conditions. The mean percent correct under
related auditory cue conditions was 41.8% (SD = 21.9; range =
38-77.6%). Under unrelated auditory cue conditions, the mean
percent correct was 49.8% (SD = 15.8; range = 17.4-65.5%).

Two factors may have contributed to low performance
under the auditory cue condition: 1) It may have been difficult for each subject to perceive auditory cue information
at the low +4 dB SN ratio. 2) Auditory cues which were dis-
similar from the white noise masker were readily incorporated
into the speech perception task. Cues such as a piano chord,
and fire alarm were not confused with the white noise, however, vacuum cleaner and bus motor noise seemed to be generally undifferentiated from the background noise according to
some subjects.

One observation reached at this point was that there
appeared to be a difference in visual speech perception which
was related to degree of visual cue relevance. The clinical
implication is that visual communication training might incorporate activities which progress from highly familiar relevant to less familiar non-relevant visual cues to prepare
the elderly adult for improved communication under less pre-
dictable everyday conditions.

A second observation supports research demonstrating
that though elderly adults may demonstrate similar pure tone
audiogram configurations, speech reception thresholds and
speech discrimination scores, their ability to perceive auditory cues in noise may vary widely under low signal-to-noise
conditions. The clinical implication is that auditory training in noise can not be based on pre-determined signal-to-
noise levels. Each level must be determined individually.

Influence of Reasoning Strategy on Speechreading Sentences
With Situational Cues

Observation of subject responses to these speechreading tasks suggested that different reasoning strategies were

being used to integrate visible speech and situational cue
information. Some subjects analyzed every observable detail
to develop their perception of the message. Other subjects
synthesized the meaning of the message from the overall situation. Since there is some question about the relative
efficiency of various reasoning procedures in a speechreading
task, two common strategies, deductive and inductive reasoning were studied (Garstecki and O'Neill, 1978) and termed
"successive scanning" and "conservative focusing" after
Bruner, Goodnow, and Austin (1956). It was hypothesized that
speechreading performance using situational cues related to
key words in a sentence would be greater when the less-
analytical, successive scanning strategy is used.

Twenty-four normal hearing and minimally hearing impaired adults ranging in age from 32 to 65 years ($\overline{X}$ = 46.5
years) served as subjects for this study. Each subject
demonstrated better ear pure tone threshold average of $\leq$ 55
dB HL (re: ANSI, 3.6 - 1969); binaural speech reception
threshold of $\leq$ 45 dB: binaural sound field discrimination
of $\geq$ 80%; binocular visual acuity of 20/40 or better; and,
normal language and visual processing skills. None had had
a lipreading class or aural rehabilitation.

Test material consisted of items selected from the
CID Everyday Speech Sentence lists which could be portrayed
visually or auditorily, such as, "I don't know what's wrong
with the car, but it won't start." Sentence presentation was
recorded in the video mode only, in the same manner as described in earlier experiments. Thus on the completed test
tape, each sentence was presented in the context of a visual
and auditory background which provided the situational cue.

Situational cues were matched with sentences and two
lists of sentence-cue items were generated. Each list included sentences matched with:

a) related visual and unrelated auditory cues, i.e.,
'The water is too cold for swimming' was presented
with a swimming pool background scene and the sound
of chirping birds.

b) related auditory and unrelated visual cues, i.e.,
'Did you forget to shut off the water?' was presented with a movie theater background scene and the
sound of running tap water.

c) unrelated visual and auditory cues, i.e., 'If we
don't get rain soon, we'll have no grass.' was

presented with a factory background scene and the
sound of trotting horses.

In addition, three sentences matched with related visual and
unrelated auditory cues and three matched with unrelated
visual and related auditory cues, served as model sentences
under the conservative focusing strategy only.

Subjects viewed the videotaped sentences in a sound-
treated audiometric test room on a 19 inch playback monitor
screen. Room lighting was controlled to optimize viewing
conditions. Practice items were used to introduce the subject to the task as well as to allow each subject to self-
adjust the playback monitor to a most comfortable listening
level for auditory cue reception.

Test sentences were presented under each strategy
condition. Under the successive scanning strategy there is,
by definition, uncertainty about the relationship between the
situation and the topic of conversation. For example, two
men speaking in front of a coffee shop as an emergency vehi-
cle siren passes in the distance may be talking about a topic
related to the coffee shop, emergency or a matter completely
unrelated to the scene. Using a successive scanning strategy, the speechreader scans and synthesizes all observable
information in his perception of the message. In this study,
subjects were instructed to view each sentence with both situational cues and re-state the sentence to the examiner. No
further instructions were provided. The subject used whatever visible speech and situational cues he felt facilitated
overall message perception.

The alternate strategy, conservative focusing, is
more circumscribed and assures that a strong relationship
exists between the sentence and some situational cue. In
everyday conversation, a person uses a conservative focusing
strategy when, using the same example, he assumes the topic
of conversation is related to the coffee shop background. If
his assumption is correct, his perception of the message is
reinforced and the conversation proceeds without interrup-
tion. If his assumption is incorrect, the situational cue
will not facilitate, and could inhibit, correct message perception. Under this strategy, subjects were required to
speechread a model sentence paired with either a related
visual or auditory cue. In speechreading the sentence, subjects were requested to identify the facilitating cue. Their
cue-type selection established a pattern for perception of a
subsequent block of test items. Thus, if the model sentence
was matched with a related auditory cue, in subsequent test
items the subject was instructed to consider the relatedness

of the auditory cue to sentence meaning. Unlike the successive scanning strategy where all available cues could be
gleaned for relatedness, in the conservative focusing strategy the order of consideration of each type of situational
cue was determined by the model item.

The results demonstrated improved speechreading
ability when situational cues related to each test sentence
were provided. Analysis of variance indicated that subjects
responded differently (F = 10.97; df = 1,88; p<0.01) as a
function of situational cue relatedness. A significant cue-
strategy condition interaction (F = 3.98; df = 1,88;
p<0.05) was also demonstrated. The interaction suggested
that while the related situational cues served to increase
speechreading performance, the effect was not demonstrated
under each reasoning strategy. Post-hoc analysis indicated
that the situational cues were more helpful under the conservative focusing strategy than the successive scanning
strategy. The inference from these data is that related
situational cues will enhance speechreading ability when
there is some guarantee of relationship between the spoken
message and the situational cues. This finding was unexpected and contrary to the popular "synthetic approach to
speechreading" reported by Jeffers and Barley (1971) and
others. However, it is important to interpret this finding
in terms of the population studied. Normal hearing and
hearing impaired adults served as subjects in this study,
but few, if any, could be described as hearing handicapped.

Overall Implications

Although additional research is warranted, the results of this preliminary series of investigations tends to
suggest that:

1) Situational cues enhance visual speech perception
and an average elderly adult should be able to use
situational cues as an adjunct to visual speech perception. However, some may ignore, misinterpret or
be distracted by situational cue information and may
require training to use these cues in everyday
communication.

2) Situational cues vary in their relatedness to the
topic of a sentence or conversation. An effort must
be made to measure the degree of topic and cue

relatedness before incorporating the use of cues in assessment and remediation of visual speech perception skill.

3) Ability to use auditory cues in visual speech perception cannot be predicted from a routine audiological test battery. Use of auditory cues with the elderly should take into account each individual's ability to perceive, and discriminate each type of cue under various noise conditions.

4) Sentence materials used for assessment and/or remediation of visual speech perception skill should be evaluated for key word visibility as well as for topic familiarity to the viewer.

5) Elderly adults may use a variety of reasoning strategies in visual speech perception with situational cues. For the beginning speechreader with a mild to moderate hearing loss, a strategy which guarantees some relationship between the idea of a message and observable situational cue may yield the greatest amount of success.

6) Age appears to be a major factor to consider when determining one's ability to benefit from situational cues in visual speech perception. The older speechreader may be less likely to be able to readily use all available information to understand a message.

These preliminary observations suggest that the audiologist should evaluate and may need to train the elderly adult to use situational cues as an adjunct to speechreading. Communication problems stemming from the auditory confusion suffered by many of the presbycusic population (Yarington, 1976) may be lessened somewhat through use of visual speech cues to compensate for and clarify message perception.

The elderly adult requires greater exposure time in message perception (Malepeai and Hutchinson, 1977). Decreasing visual acuity (Botwinick, 1973) and visual accommodation time (Weiss, 1959), along with greater rigidity in interpersonal communication suggests the need for taking advantage of as much relevant information as possible to effect successful interpersonal communication. Increasing the

chances for successful communication should decrease the
elderly person's anxiety and may increase their motivation
to communicate with others.

REFERENCES

1. American National Standards Institute, Specifications
    for Audiometers. ANSI S3.6 - 1969. New York:
    American National Standards Institute, 1970.

2. American Speech and Hearing Association, Issues in
    Ethics. *ASHA, 19,* 343, 1977.

3. Botwinick, J., Aging and Behavior. New York:
    Springer, 1973.

4. Bruner, J. S., Goodnow, J. J., and Austin, G. A., A
    Study of Thinking. New York, N.Y.: John Wiley
    and Sons, Inc., 1956.

5. Davis, H., and Silverman, S. R., Hearing and Deafness.
    New York: Holt, Rinehart and Winston, Inc., 1968.

6. Fleming, M., A total approach to communication therapy.
    J. Acad. Rehab. Aud., 5, 28-31, 1972.

7. Garstecki, D., Situational cues in visual speech
    perception. *J. Amer. Aud. Soc., 2,* 99-106, 1976.

8. Garstecki, D., and O'Neill, J., Situational cue and
    strategy influence on speechreading. Unpublished
    manuscript, 1978.

9. Jeffers, J., and Barley, M., Speechreading (Lipreading).
    Springfield, Ill.: Charles C. Thomas, Inc. 1971.

10. Malepeai, B. and Hutchinson, J., Word retrieval and
    visual processing skills among the elderly. Paper
    presented at the Annual Convention of the American
    Speech and Hearing Association, Chicago, 1977.

11. Morkovin, B., and Moore, L., Life-Situation Speechreading
    Through the Cooperation of Senses. Los Angeles, CA:
    University of Southern Press, 1944.

12. Nielson, B., Measurement of visual speech comprehension.
    J. Speech Hear. Res., 13, 856-860, 1970.

13. Utley, J., A test of lipreading ability. J. Speech
    Hear. Dis., 11, 109-116, 1946.

14. Wales, J., Garstecki, D., and Privratsky, K., Assessment
    of the aged adult's ability to use everyday communi-
    cation cues. Paper presented at the Annual Convention
    of the American Speech and Hearing Association,
    Chicago, IL, 1977.

15. Weiss, A., Sensory functions. In J. E. Birren (eds.)
    Handbook of Aging and the Individual: Psychological
    and Biological Aspects. Chicago: University of
    Chicago Press, 1959.

16. Yarington, C., Jr. Presbycusis. In J. Northern (ed.),
    Hearing Disorders. Boston: Little, Brown, 1976.

Chapter 8

The Effects of Age on the Visual
Perception of Speech

CARL A. BINNIE, PH. D.

With the increased attention the entire area of gerontology is receiving, it is becoming obvious that there can
be profound effects on the elderly person's physical, psychological and social well-being. Audiologists are becoming
more cognizant of the psycho-social effects associated with
communication problems among the aged and are assuming increased responsibility for the auditory rehabilitation of
this population. They are aware of the possibility of overall neural atrophy of the auditory system and its effect on
communication performance. As a result, audiologists are
establishing programs for the independent living aged person
and are finding a place on the total patient management team
in health care facilities, retirement and nursing homes. In-
service workshops for nurses and other para-medical personnel
are part of the rehabilitation process designed to teach
others about the effects of hearing impairment and how to
modify the environment to improve communication efficiency
for this population.

Visual communication is an important part of the
aural rehabilitation process because speechreading, as well
as environmental and situational cues, may improve communication, particularly for those who experience a reduction in
the amount of information received through the auditory
channel. Several studies have demonstrated that auditory and
visual cues interact to produce an increase in intelligibility on the order of 20% over that which the auditory system alone might be able to decode (Binnie, 1973; Binnie,
1974; Erber, 1969; Erber, 1972.).

While it is known that the aged person frequently
demonstrates difficulty in auditory recognition of speech,
relatively little is known about the effects of age on the
visual perception of speech. It is likely that the over-all
visual perceptual performance decreases with age. If this is
the case, then the audiologist must be aware of these deficits as they may influence the nature of the rehabilitation

program. In order to understand the effects of age on the
visual communication of speech, we need to direct our attention to: 1) the relationship between visual acuity and
speechreading, 2) the effect of age on the speechreading process, 3) the prevalence of visual pathology among aged persons and 4) the influence of perceptual processing, including
learning, memory and motivation for this group of adults.

Very little information is available concerning the
nature of visual perception within the aging population.
However, some experimental evidence suggests that visual perception may be an age related process, i.e., speechreading
ability decreases as chronological age increases (Farrimond,
1959; Goetzinger, 1963; Ewertsen and Nielsen, 1971). While
the precise reasons for this reduction do not appear to be
fully understood, research associated with visual acuity and
central processing has shown depreciation of these functions
as an inverse correlate with age (Cowdry, 1939; Dublin,
1967). Whether changes in speechreading ability as a function of advancing age are the result of physiological or
psychological effects upon the older individual still remains
unanswered.

Sanders (1971) reported that there are two periods in
life when visual problems are most likely to occur. These
are during early school years and during adulthood. These
are the same periods when hearing impairment is most preva-
lent. Thus, loss of vision can have pronounced effects on
the auditory-visual comprehension of speech. For the elderly, the onset of visual loss may be slow and the amount of
deterioration may be marked before the person recognizes it
as a problem. Just as the person learns to compensate for
insidious loss of hearing, he compensates for visual loss
through adaptive behavior. He may reject his need for a
hearing aid or glasses. In fact, the visual difficulty may
only be evident during those times when the person with a
hearing loss is forced to rely on visual cues for
communication.

Experimental evidence suggests that age, especially
beyond middle-age, is an important factor in determining
visual perceptual performance in that speechreading tends to
decrease as age increases (Farrimond, 1959; Ewertsen and
Nielsen, 1971). Visual acuity does appear to be a variable
in the analysis of visual perception since peripheral impairment of the visual system will tend to reduce recognition and
comprehension. Lovering and Hardick (1969) and Hardick, Oyer
and Irion (1970) showed that speechreading performance de-
clined as visual acuity decreased beyond 20/40. In addition,
Erber (1974) has shown that there is a significant effect on

the individual's speechreading ability regarding the angle,
distance and illumination of the speaker's face.

One of the problems confronting the audiologist is
determining who needs speechreading training. In an attempt
to establish baseline data which is representative of average
performance for a wide array of linguistic materials, Binnie
(1976) proposed a speechreading profile for the assessment
of visual speech perception. It was felt that this profile
might span the analytic-synthetic continuum and assist in the
measurement of basic visual speech perception. It also may
help determine the type and nature of the speechreading
training program and serve as a guide to compare pre- and
post-treatment training leading to criterion performance
levels. However, it is known that experimental variables
such as the nature of stimulus materials, speaker differences, recording and testing conditions, as well as hearing
status, visual acuity and age are all highly relevant considerations that could singularly affect visual comprehension of
speech.

Visual Perception Within the Aging Population

In an investigation using a sample of 180 industrial
workers between 20 and 65 years of age, Farrimond (1959)
found that the optimal age for visual perception occurred
before age 39. In fact, Farrimond found that scores dimin-
ished at a rate of approximately 8% per decade beyond age 40.
Farrimond concluded that differences in speechreading performance among various age groups did not occur from a decreased ability to learn speechreading. Instead, he hypothesized that age related changes occurred as a function of an
individual's ability to deal efficiently with the visual
information which was available. Farrimond suggested that
older hearing-impaired individuals may pay greater attention
than younger persons to lip movements and facial expressions
when attending to speech and proposed that the decrease in
visual perception was due to aging effects upon the central
processes involved in perception of speech through the visual
mode.

Farrimond explained the speechreading process as a
form of statistical correlation between visual and auditory
patterns with the number of potential alternatives from which
selection is made being limited by the presence of contextual
information. According to Farrimond, the aging individual
has difficulty in forming concepts with the concept formation
process being particularly impaired in situations regarding
decision speed.

Goetzinger (1963) found a significant negative association between age and visual perception utilizing the
Utley Sentence Test. Goetzinger investigated the speechreading performances of 36 normally-hearing subjects with an age
range of 18 to 37 for comparison of monocular versus binocular vision. Although the investigation was not designed to
assess the relationship between age and visual perception
skills, Goetzinger inadvertently found that speechreading
performance for sentence materials was poorer among older
subjects (age range 25 to 37 years) than for younger ones
(age range 18 to 22 years). Goetzinger concluded that subtle
changes, which have a deleterious effect on the visual perception of speech, take place after age 25. However, the
origin of these changes, whether psychological or physiological, could not be determined from his data.

Ewertsen and Nielsen (1971) found that auditory,
auditory-visual and visual scores for a word recognition task
progressively decreased as a function of age. They found
that with a signal-to-noise ratio of -20 dB, the auditory
scores revealed a complete masking of speech. Auditory-
visual scores at this signal-to-noise ratio showed that correct perception of the stimulus words occurred 50% of the
time. Ewertsen and Nielsen attributed this improvement under
auditory-visual conditions to vision or speechreading in
noise. Analysis of the scores obtained under visual-only
conditions yielded a much larger reduction in perceptual performance than scores obtained under the auditory-visual
condition. When comparing these results, utilizing the three
conditions discussed above, among the three age groups
tested (20, 50, and 70 year olds), it became evident that
deterioration of perception paralleled advancing age.

Pelson and Prather (1974) examined the effects of age
and hearing impairment upon two different types of speechreading tasks. In this experiment, Pelson and Prather divided a total of 36 subjects into three groups of 12 persons,
which differed primarily on the basis of age and auditory
status. The first group consisted of young normally-hearing
subjects who were 19 to 26 years of age, the second group
contained older normally-hearing subjects between the ages
of 52 to 61, and the third group was comprised of older
hearing-impaired individuals who were 51 to 59 years old.
The mean duration of hearing loss for the hearing-impaired
group was 10.7 years and all individuals in this group exhibited bilateral sensorineural hearing impairments of 50 dB
(ANSI, 1969) or greater for the better ear. All 36 subjects
viewed two lists of sentences from the John Tracy Lip Reading
Test, recorded on black and white video tape under two

experimental speechreading conditions. Specifically, the
first list was presented in a visual-only format while the
second list was given under the condition visual-with-con-
straints, in which appropriate message-related 35 mm color
slides were shown just before the speaker delivered the
sentence. Under both these conditions, the subjects were
permitted to view the stimulus item twice, i.e., once at a 0
degree and once at a 45 degree azimuth.

The results of the Pelson and Prather study showed
that absolute visual speech perception for sentences measured
under a visual-only condition was better among younger normally-hearing individuals (19 to 26 years) than for older
normally-hearing subjects (52 to 61 years) or hearing-
impaired persons (51 to 59 years). However, among the two
older groups, hearing-impaired subjects performed slightly
better than normally-hearing individuals. Under the related
message speechreading condition, older hearing-impaired persons showed greater improvement than either the younger or
older normally-hearing subjects. Pelson and Prather specu-
lated that hearing-impairment rather than age determined the
extent to which visual constraints were used in speechreading
since hearing-impaired subjects benefited more through the
use of related-message pictures than did normally-hearing
subjects. But, regardless of the presence or absence of
message-related cues, the effect of age upon visual perception performance for sentence material was evident from the
data included in their investigation.

Shoop and Binnie (1978) investigated the effects of
age on the visual perception of speech by using two types of
stimulus materials, consonant vowel (CV) syllables and CID
Everyday Speech Sentences. The first set of stimuli included
100 items in which five randomizations of each of 20 CV
syllables were presented. This was a test of viseme cate-
gorization as described by Binnie, Jackson and Montgomery in
1976. This test was selected because the 1976 study by
Binnie et al. represented a set of normative data obtained
from young normally hearing subjects and because the test
results represented a means by which specific error patterns
could be analyzed. However, it was not known whether the
set of normative data for young normally hearing subjects
could be applied to a group of older subjects. The second
set of stimuli (i.e., sentences) was selected to determine if
visual speech performance at the syllable level generalized
to visual perception ability at the sentence level.

A sample of 110 adult subjects was selected from the
normally hearing population of those persons seen at the
Purdue University Hearing Clinic. All subjects met the

criterion of 1) normal auditory sensitivity (500, 1000 and
2000 Hz at 25 dB (ANSI, 1969) for the better ear), 2) normal
visual acuity (normal or corrected binocular vision to 20/40
or better as tested by the Snellen Eye Chart) and 3) age
(four specific age decade groups). There were 30 subjects in
each of the decade groups 40-50 years, 51-60 years and 61-70
years. There were 20 subjects in the group 71 years old or
greater. This group was limited to a smaller number because
of the imposed normally-hearing criterion. None of the 110
subjects had any previous lipreading instruction.

All subjects in the four age decade groups who participated in this study were given the Consonant Confusion
Lipreading Test (Binnie, Jackson and Montgomery, 1976) and
List 2 of the CID Everyday Speech Sentences (revised by Hood
and Dixon, 1969). These tests were counter-balanced among
the testing sessions so that one half of the participants
viewed the consonant-vowel stimuli first and the sentence
material last and one half of the subjects viewed this testing format in reverse order. In addition, all subjects were
randomly assigned to viewing sessions in groups of eight,
irrespective of age and sex. Finally, all subjects were
asked to repeat aloud six sentences of varying syllable
length, selected from Lists 3 and 4 of the Revised CID Everyday Speech Sentences (Hood and Dixon, 1969) and recorded on a
Language Master (Bell and Howell, Model 711 B1) in order to
demonstrate adequate short term auditory memory.

The two types of lipreading stimuli were presented
from a video-tape closed circuit television monitor arrangement using the same talker. This black and white video-taped
life size image of the speaker was presented in a front
facing position.

Table 1 shows the mean scores and standard deviations
of the four age categories for total test performance for the
CV stimuli. The mean scores for the age ranges 40-50, 51-60,
and 61-70 years were similar. However, the 71+ year old
group showed a reduced lipreading score. An analysis of
variance revealed statistically significant differences as a
function of age with Treatment 4 (71+ year old group) being
significantly different from all other treatments. There
were no differences among individuals between the ages of
40-70 years.

When comparing the visual perception of CV syllables
for the aged persons to the normative data from the Binnie,
Jackson and Montgomery (1976) study, it was noted that the
40-50 year old group met criterion performance for eight of
nine viseme categories. The 51-60 and 61-70 year old groups
failed to meet criterion for two viseme categories and the

TABLE 1

Mean scores and standard deviations for total test performances derived from four age categories. Data are from 110 observers with the total possible score being 95.

			Total Test Performances		
Treatment		1	2	3	4
Age Range		40 to 50 years	51 to 60 years	61 to 70 years	$\geq$ 71 years
$\overline{X}$ =		72.50	67.30	71.40	59.60
S.D. =		13.00	14.70	10.60	12.60
N =		30	30	30	20

129

oldest group (71+ years) were below criterion for seven
viseme categories. These results are shown in Table 2.

The final portion of this investigation was concerned
with an analysis of the relationship between visual perceptual performances for consonant-vowel syllables and CID sentences. This included the study of the effect of chronological age upon the visual speech perception for sentence
material.

For the purpose of determining whether age was a factor influencing the visual perceptual performances of sentences, lipreading scores, representing percent correct recognition from List 2 of the revised CID Sentences, were obtained
from five age treatments (20-87 years). The data are shown
in Table 3.

Statistical analysis of these five age groups revealed significant differences as a function of increasing age.
The youngest group was significantly better in the visual
perception of sentences than all four older decade groups.
The observers in this youngest group demonstrated an average
speechreading score of 37.4% (S.D. = 11.80). Scores for the
four older treatments deteriorated in a step-wise fashion as
age increased. Scores for the 40-50 year old group averaged
26.4% (S.D. = 12.00), the 51-60 year old group averaged 23.6%
(S.D. = 13.00) and the 61-70 year old group scored 18.5%
(S.D. = 10.00). The oldest group was poorest in speechreading performance with a mean score of 13.50 (S.D. = 8.40).
When comparing the middle three age treatments (40-50, 51-60
and 61-70), results indicated that the 40-50 year olds and
51-60 year olds performed similarly. However, the 61-70 year
old group was significantly different from the 40-50 year
olds and the 51-60 year olds. The 71+ year old group was
significantly different from all the younger groups.

The mean performance levels for sentences, when compared to CV syllable performances, showed a more consistent
decline as age increased. Figure 1 shows a histogram with
the mean performances for CV syllables and CID Sentences for
five age groups. The differences among the mean sentence
scores revealed a rate of decline by age decade that favor-
ably supported Farrimond's (1959) findings. More specifically, sentence speechreading ability decreased consistently
across age decades. Sentences seem to be a more sensitive
measure of age-related effects on the visual speech perception process than viseme categories within CV syllables, although consistent age effects were shown using both of these
syllables.

The findings in the present study were in general
agreement with previous experimental results which have shown

TABLE 2

The mean scores obtained from Treatments 1, 2, 3, and 4 for total test performance and nine viseme categories are marked according to whether they were equal to and above (+) or below (–) the criterion levels established by Binnie, Jackson, and Montgomery (1976) at –1 standard deviation from the mean.

Normative Data (Binnie, et al., 1976)	Total Test	fv	pbm	w	ln	∫ʒ	r	θð	tdsz	kg
Mean Score	78.60	9.60	14.20	4.60	8.60	8.20	4.10	7.70	14.80	6.70
Criterion Level (–1 S.D.)	71.50	9.10	13.30	3.90	7.00	4.70	2.90	6.10	11.90	4.20
Treatment 1 40 to 50 Years Mean Score	72.50 +	9.40 +	13.80 +	4.40 +	8.40 +	7.70 +	2.60 –	8.20 +	13.70 +	4.30 +
Treatment 2 51 to 60 Years Mean Score	67.30 +	9.30 +	13.70 +	4.10 +	7.80 +	6.10 +	2.40 –	7.80 +	12.80 +	3.20 –
Treatment 3 61 to 70 Years Mean Score	71.40 –	9.80 +	14.00 +	4.50 +	7.70 +	8.10 +	2.40 –	7.70 +	14.40 +	2.90 –
Treatment 4 ≥71 Years Mean Score	59.40 –	9.10 +	13.10 –	3.60 –	6.40 –	6.60 +	1.40 –	5.40 –	11.20 –	2.60 –

TABLE 3

Mean scores and standard deviations for percent correct performance derived from five age treatments when presented with List 2 of the CID Everyday Speech Sentences. Data are from 140 observers with a total possible score being 100%.

			Mean Total Test Performance % Correct			
Treatment	Young Normals	1	2	3	4
Age Range	20 to 23	40 to 50	51 to 60	61 to 70	71
$\bar{X}$ =	37.40	26.40	23.60	18.50	13.50
S.D. =	11.80	12.00	13.00	10.00	8.40
N =	30	30	30	30	20

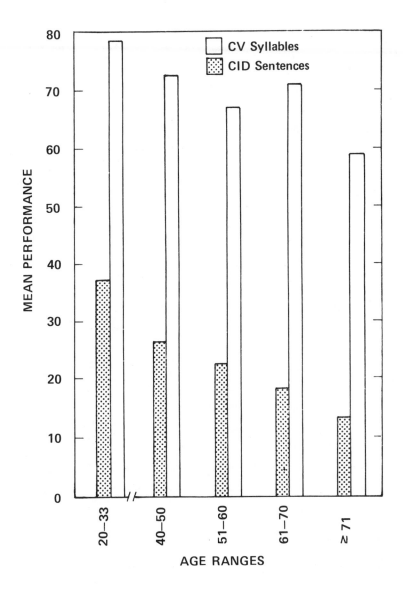

FIG. 1. *Histogram comparing distributions of mean performance for CV syllables and CID Sentences among five age treatments.*

a negative correlation between chronological age and speed-reading ability (Farrimond, 1959; Goetzinger, 1963; Ewertsen and Nielsen, 1971; Pelson and Prather, 1974). Using numbers and sentences with relevant background scenes, Farrimond reported that speechreading ability decreased at an approximate rate of 8% per decade among the age groups above the age of 39. Ewertsen and Nielsen (1971) found that an approximate 10% decrease in speechreading performance occurred among 50 and 70 year olds using a word recognition task in a visual-only condition. It should be noted that these investigations utilized different sets of stimulus materials, i.e., numbers, words, and sentences, and that these types of test materials could possibly reflect a more sensitive measure to speech-reading ability as a function of advancing age than visual perception of consonant-vowel syllables.

Whether or not age related effects upon the visual perception of speech can be attributed to physiological or psychological factors cannot be determined from the present investigation. However, research evidence concerned with presbycusis refers to an overall general neural atrophy which may effect auditory speech processing ability (Schuknecht, 1964). In a similar way, Farrimond commented on the visual correlate of age and speechreading scores. He stated that, "It may be that the older man with a hearing defect may pay more attention to lip movements and facial expression when listening to speech and that the decline in ability as indicated by the speechreading test is due to aging of the central process involved in this activity" (1959, p. 188). Farrimond (1959) also attributed changes in selection and decision speeds in the concept formation processes as a "true aging difficulty" (1959, p. 189). Since these central processes are thought to be part of the speechreading process, Farrimond concluded that the effect of age upon the visual perception of speech was centrally oriented.

There is some experimental evidence to support age related effects upon the senescense of cell tissue in the human brain. Dublin (1967) stated that senile changes of the nervous system are similar to those found elsewhere throughout the body. Age produces cerebral atrophy as well as degeneration of dermal elastic tissue. In general, no part of the brain escapes atrophy, but this tends to be more pronounced in the frontal region, less in the temporal, and even less in the parietal and occipital regions, cerebellum and the brain stem. The cortex shows a general thinning; nerve cell loss is constant as a function of age. In addition, cortical cell layers become disorganized. Among the surviving nerve cells, the degree of degeneration varies greatly

regarding the type and stage of cell destruction. Dublin
(1967) reported that the degree of alteration of nerve tissue
in senility roughly parallels advancing age. Such neuropath-
ological evidence as this supports the notion that the deleterious effects of aging on the speechreading process may
occur due to central involvement. Since cell degeneration
is found uniformly throughout the brain as a whole, it seems
logical to conclude that those central processes which are
associated with the visual perception of speech may be less
efficient in the geriatric individual.

Visual Pathology Due to the Aging Process

The aging process is viewed by some to be a general
part of the development of life. However, others strike a
difference between development and aging. They view development as those changes leading to adaptive behavior and
aging as those changes which are de-adaptive and reduce the
ability of the individual to survive. According to Anderson
(1964), aging refers to those changes which result in a decrement of function after the long stable period of middle
age.
During the aging process there is tremendous individual variability related to the pattern, onset and rate of
change. This individual variation tends to be influenced by
inherited characteristics and by environmental factors.
Birren (1964) suggested that environmental factors may be
more important influences of general physical deterioration
associated with the aging organism. We can appreciate this
with our understanding of the overall deterioration in auditory functioning as a result of the aging process. The
auditory system is not the only sensory system which shows
declining sensitivity with advancing age; this is the case of
most sensory systems including the visual system. According
to Kalish (1977, p. 52), "Most persons over age 60 must adapt
to some type of sensory change that reduces the amount of
information he receives from his environment".
Statistics related to the incidence of hearing loss
as a result of age suggest that the rate of hearing impairment during the period from 20-75 years increases from
13/1000 to about 399/1000 (Metropolitan Life Insurance Co.;
U.S. Health Interview Survey, 1976). Between the ages of
60-80 years this rate accelerates to about 250/1000. Thus,
about one of four aged persons has a significant hearing impairment. In this same age range, about 80/1000 are blind
(Kalish, 1977). It is estimated that approximately 400,000
persons in the U.S. are legally blind - defined as vision

20/200 or poorer in the better eye with corrective lenses
(Pitorak, 1971, p. 1076). Birren (1964), Weale (1965) and
Botwinick (1973) have all reported that there is generally
little change in visual acuity during the period from 15-50
years. However, it is not uncommon to see sharp declines in
visual acuity after age 50 and poor vision among persons 70
years of age is generally expected. The causes of visual
deterioration among the aged may be related to 1) external
changes of the eye, 2) alterations in the condition of the
lens, and 3) intra-ocular conditions. Moreover, problems in
visual perceptual performance such as reduced visual memory,
retention and response time may contribute to the overall
reduction in visual and auditory-visual speech comprehension.

Visual Acuity and Aging

        Basic tests of visual performance are reviewed by
Schow et al. (1978). One of the most common tests of visual
adequacy is the measure of visual acuity. This test measures
the smallest object which can be perceived at a given distance. Accommodation is another indication of visual sensory
integrity. This test measures the ability of the eye to focus on objects at different distances. Another indicator of
visual efficiency is dark adaptation. This is defined as the
time it takes to reach maximum acuity in the dark and the
acuity level finally reached. Depth perception (stereopsis)
is associated with binocularity and a problem here interferes
with spatial orientation. In severe cases this may result in
double vision, or diplopia.
        According to Weiss (1959), Birren (1964) and Botwin-
ick (1973), those aspects of vision which deteriorate with
advancing age are changes in the required illumination level,
contrast discrimination, color vision and critical flicker
fusion.
        Those conditions causing deterioration of vision in
the aged are of several different varieties and can be divided into functional changes, senile tissue degeneration and
distinct pathologic conditions (Sanders and Smith, 1971).
Aging changes in the eyes appear in the late 30's or early
40's with the development of presbyopia, the aging eye. This
is probably one of the earliest manifestations of the modification of vision associated with age. The presbyopic eye is
unable to focus from far to near vision. People with presbyopia frequently have difficulty seeing fine print at a near
distance point. To compensate for this alteration of the
near point of accommodation, these people hold reading

material at arm's length (Pitorak, 1971; Sanders and Smith, 1971; and Kalish, 1977).

Sanders and Smith (1971) indicated that older lens fibers migrate toward the center of the lens where they become more dense and rigid, affecting the curvature of the lens. Because of this modification the lens becomes more resistant to change by action of the ciliary muscle. Presbyopia can be treated with corrective lenses, thereby restoring the power of accommodation. Presbyopia may not affect distance vision, but it may necessitate a biconvex lens for reading comfort. In many cases, the elderly have bifocal lenses for correction of both near and far vision. If the near point continues to slip, stronger reading glasses may well be needed over the next two decades (Sanders and Smith, 1971).

External Changes of the Eye

While it does not profoundly affect vision, senile atrophy of the various tissues surrounding the eyeball is characteristic of the aging process. This causes a distinct change in the facial appearance. The tissues of the lids become atrophic and the lids sunken with drooping of the eyelids. Changes in the skin and musculature may appear in the form of characteristic crow's feet. Sanders and Smith (1971) further reported that alterations of the muscle tonus in the eyelid can result in a spastic up-turning of the lower lid. This is called senile entropion. Occasional changes in the musculature may cause the lower lid to evert (ectropion). Finally, the eyelids may be subject to tumors of the skin, a condition encountered more frequently in the elderly patient. According to Sanders and Smith (1971), benign tumors, suborrheic keratoses, cutaneous horns, keratin cysts and basal cell carcinoma are common neoplasms of the eyelids increasing with age.

Conditions Involving the Lens

As reported earlier, presbyopia is a common condition among elderly persons. This is basically a lens problem resulting from new lens fibers migrating toward the area of the equatorial region and gradually forming a dense central nucleus (Sanders and Smith, 1971).

According to Sanders (1971), lens problems are usually reflected in abnormalities of visual acuity and the ability of the eye to distinguish fine details. The finer

the detailed work required by the eyes, the greater are the
illumination needs.

Another factor which determines the eye's capability
to do detailed work is related to the angle at which the
light strikes the retina. Visual acuity is also affected by
the distance between the eye and the object being observed;
the greater the separation, the poorer visual acuity becomes.
Decreases in visual acuity may be grouped under three refrac-
tive error hearings: 1) myopia (nearsightedness), 2) hyperopia (farsightedness) and 3) astigmatism (distorted vision).

Myopia is an abnormal elongation of the shape of the
eyeball. Light rays emanating from distant objects come into
focus at a point before they reach the retina. Thus, the
image of distant objects is blurred while near vision remains
unimpaired.

Hyperopia results from a shorter than normal distance
between the cornea and retina. Thus the visual image remains
out of focus by the time the light waves reach the retina.
To compensate for this loss of focus, the ciliary muscles
must contract strongly to control the shape and thickness of
the lens. Because of the dense lens fitness in the presbyopic eye, visual accommodation cannot be achieved without
corrective lenses.

Astigmatism is an irregularity in the curve of the
cornea resulting in an uneven focusing of light rays from the
same source. For one with astigmatism, objects appear fuzzy,
elongated or flattened. Astigmatism may occur alone or in
combination with myopia and hyperopia.

Cataracts

A cataract is defined as any opacity of the lens.
It is "a cloudiness of the lens of the eye which blocks the
normal passage of light rays through the pupil to the retina"
(Public Health Service Publication No. 793, 1963). There are
many causes of cataracts, including 1) congenital problems,
2) direct trauma, 3) radiation, 4) intra-ocular inflammatory
disease and 5) senile cataract (Sanders and Smith, 1971,
p. 327).

While cataracts can occur at any age, the majority
occur in the older age group as a result of aging and degeneration. The most common type of cataracts are senile cataracts. They are present in most persons over age 60
(Pitorak, 1971). Sanders and Smith (1971) reported that by
age 80 every individual probably has some lenticular opacity.
Anderson (1971) reported that at the age of 80, 85% of all
persons have some opacity.

Senile cataracts fall into one of two large categories: 1) cortical cataracts and 2) nuclear cataracts (Sanders
and Smith, 1971). The exact cause of cortical cataract is
not understood, but it may be the result of a matabolic
change in the lens fibers that causes degenerative changes.
The nuclear cataract is an exaggeration of the ordinary physiologic accumulation of the central lens fibers. The nucleus
can produce a pronounced distortion of the image on the
retina, with accompanying visual loss (Sanders and Smith,
1971).

The progress of cataract development varies from
person to person. The onset is usually gradual, signalled or
blurred vision or a hazy appearance. The effect on visual
acuity will be determined by the area of opacification with
peripheral opaqueness of the lens not affecting visual
acuity greatly (Pitorak, 1971). Cataracts characteristically
affect distance vision, particularly when the condition becomes progressive and opacity becomes more diffuse affecting
the pupil area of the lens. There is little therapeutic
treatment for cataracts except surgical extraction, and in
many cases the patient's vision is restored (Sanders and
Smith, 1971).

Intra-ocular Conditions

Intra-ocular conditions can involve the retina,
choroid, and optic nerve, as well as the cornea, lens and
vitrous body (Sanders and Smith, 1971). The most important
group of conditions occurring in the retina and the choroid
are those caused by vascular disease. The retina is a frequent site of study of systemic vascular changes such as
arteriosclerosis. Hardening and thickening of the arterial
walls can cause occlusion of the central vein or artery
causing sudden, almost complete loss of vision (Sanders and
Smith, 1971).

Vascular alterations of the choroid are clinically
significant when present in the area of the macula. The area
of central vision is the fovea centralis and includes a small
amount of surrounding retina known as the macula. This area
is completely void of retinal circulation and therefore receives all its nutrition from the underlying capillary layer
of the choroid (Sanders and Smith, 1971). Arteriosclerotic
changes in the capillary layer of the choroid are probably
the main source of visual deterioration in the aged. This is
referred to as senile macular degeneration.

Other retinal disorders resulting from systemic diseases include 1) hypertensive and renal retinopathy,

2) rheumatoid arthritis, 3) anemia, and 4) diabetes. Retinal
damage is often permanent and not amenable to treatment. In
addition, there may be a mild reduction of visual acuity
caused by arteriosclerotic optic atrophy. This is caused by
changes in the small nutrient arteries entering the optic
nerve from the surrounding optic nerve sheaths. Sudden
massive loss of vision, usually bilateral, may be seen in the
elderly patient from optic nerve involvement in temporal
arteritis (Sanders and Smith, 1971).

Glaucoma

        Glaucoma is a condition of the eye characterized by
increased intra-ocular pressure leading to cupping and degeneration of the optic disk and changes in the visual field
(Pitorak, 1971). According to Sanders and Smith (1971),
glaucoma may be grouped into several varieties: 1) congenital glaucoma, 2) secondary to trauma and 3) intra-ocular
diseases such as tumor, vascular disease and inflammation.
Glaucoma is the eye disease most important from the stand-
point of loss of vision although cataracts are frequently
seen.
        Glaucoma seldom occurs in people under age 35 but is
one of the greatest enemies to vision loss in older people.
Anderson (1971), Pitorak (1971) and Sanders (1971) all reported that early symptoms of glaucoma occur in the late 40's,
with approximately 2% of the population having this disease.
Glaucoma accounts for approximately 12% of all blindness in
the United States.
        The onset of glaucoma is usually insidious with loss
of peripheral vision present before other symptoms. There is
an increased loss of peripheral field before the central
visual fields are affected. The disease usually begins in
one eye but if left untreated can affect binocular vision.
There is no cure for glaucoma; treatment is usually directed
toward reducing intra-ocular tension and keeping it at a safe
level. This may arrest progression of the disease (Anderson,
1971).
        The importance of establishing and maintaining good
visual adequacy for purposes of contact with one's physical
and social life space is obvious. The concern with the visual aspect of communication stems from the important role
that vision plays for a hearing impaired person as a result
of an inability to perceive the auditory signal completely.
        The aging process tends to cause a slow but steady
decrease in visual efficiency. Many of these processes are
distinct physiologic and pathologic events while others are

local manifestations of tissue degeneration seen elsewhere in
the body (Sanders and Smith, 1971). Many of the conditions
causing visual loss in the aged are characteristic of older
individuals but start in young persons and progress further
with increasing age; thus, early recognition is important.

Fortunately, many of the pathologic conditions discussed in this paper are related to peripheral changes and
may be corrected with appropriate refraction. Thus, referral
to various health care professionals is an important step for
those suspected of having difficulties in vision.

Summary

While some studies suggest that speechreading performance decreases as visual acuity decreases (Lovering and
Hardick, 1969; Hardick et al., 1970), others have reported
decreased speechreading ability among elderly persons even
though visual acuity was held constant within normal or near-
normal limits (Farrimond, 1959; Ewertsen and Nielsen, 1971;
Pelson and Prather, 1974; Shoop and Binnie, 1978). Visual
acuity factors may not be of primary importance in influencing performance on speechreading tasks. At least for the
elderly, special attention must be given to other factors.

It is likely that over-all visual perceptual performance diminishes with age. Schow et al. (1978) summarized
several experiments documenting the presence of visual processing difficulties among the elderly. They reported that
perceptual processing among the elderly may be reduced because of a variety of. factors.

First, because of anatomic changes in the sensory
systems, the central nervous system (CNS) may receive less
information from which to make accurate processing decisions.
Secondly, as a result of CNS alterations during aging, the
ability to integrate information from several senses or within one sense may deteriorate. Finally, aged persons may
display a rigidity in responding and a reduced ability to
alter original percepts. Age effects are usually more profound when interfering visual stimuli and reduced contrasts
are used. These factors may account for the reduction in
visual speech comprehension.

Experiments by Wallace (1956) and Riegel (1956)
suggested that older subjects required a much greater exposure time in order to identify designs, words and pictures.
In addition to greater exposure time, a series of experiments
has shown that there may be a loss of speed of response behavior as age increases. Donahue (1971) suggested that the
slowing of response may be largely central in origin rather

than the result of changes in the peripheral (sensory or motor) end organs. With the slowing of response concomitant with aging, organization of behavior becomes more difficult. Donahue (1971) suggested that when testing the elderly we should be aware that 1) examination time may need to be increased, 2) directions may not be easily comprehended, 3) the patient may require more reassurance with respect to alleviation of fears and misconceptions, 4) testing procedures may require a greater detail of instruction and 5) may need to provide ample time for written instructions or responses. These factors certainly may contribute to reduced performance among the elderly, particularly when testing and teaching speechreading skills.

It should be remembered that the visual decoding of articulatory gestures may be a difficult and frustrating task for any of us. In addition, the speechreading testing situation may be the first experience for an elderly person where he is asked to try to decode visually encoded gestures. For the elderly, this may be a stressful experience. Older adults seem to anticipate difficulties in learning; they may be apprehensive when approaching a new task. They often appear overly-cautious and may be fearful of making mistakes. Speed in learning and adaptation to new material can be a problem particularly when unlearning old habits is necessary (Donahue, 1971).

The information presented in this paper has some pertinent implications for the testing and teaching of speechreading to aged persons. Tests of speechreading should be administered using normative data to determine if older persons are able to achieve average scores. In the clinical assessment procedure the following recommendations are suggested:

1) use a standardized film (or video-tape) test of speechreading
2) check visual acuity of subjects to assure that performance is 20/40 or better
3) in case history interview, follow the prevalence of visual difficulties just as we trace auditory problems and make appropriate referrals
4) administer tests of visual-only performance as well as auditory-visual to determine how well the two senses interact
5) give ample time for directions and response behavior
6) encourage guessing behavior; they may be closer to the correct response than they think

7) inspection of results of tests of viseme categori-
   zation may provide a good basis for training in
   consonant discrimination and recognition.
8) use sentences and synthetic (environmental) cues
   which may provide a better estimate of speechreading performance than CV syllables, words or
   unrelated sentences
9) realize the frustrations of trying to speechread
   and try to increase one's motivation
10) encourage the use of environmental cues and auditory
    information to increase estimates of over-all
    intelligibility.

In conclusion, there are several factors which may
alter the visual perceptual ability of elderly persons.
These factors tend to be reflected in poorer speechreading
performance and, as a result, have implications for the
audiologist in charge of the aural rehabilitation plan. Factors such as hearing impairment, visual acuity (or other
visual problems), auditory-visual interaction, central processing problems, the nature of the stimulus-response task,
the type of stimulus materials, learning, memory and motivation may all interact to affect speechreading performance.

REFERENCES

1. Anderson, H. C., Newton's Geriatric Nursing, St. Louis:
    C. V. Mosby Co., 1971.

2. Anderson, J. E., Psychological research on changes and
    transformations during development and aging.
    Chapter in Birren, J. E. (Ed.) Relations of develop-
    ment and aging. Springfield, Ill.: Charles C.
    Thomas (1964).

3. Binnie, C. A., Auditory-visual intelligibility of
    various speech materials presented in three noise
    backgrounds. In Nielson, H. B. and Kampp, E. (Eds.).
    Visual and Audio-Visual Perception of Speech.
    Scandinavian Audiology, Suppl. 4, 255-280 (1974).

4. Binnie, C. A., Bi-sensory articulation functions for
    normal hearing and sensorineural hearing loss
    patients. *J. Acad. Rehab. Audiology, 6,* 43-53
    (1973).

5. Binnie, C. A., Relevant Aural Rehabilitation. Chapter
    in Northern, J. L. (Ed.) Hearing Disorders. Boston,
    Mass.: Little, Brown and Co. (1976).

6. Binnie, C. A., Jackson, P. L. and Montgomery, A. A.
    Visual Intelligibility of consonants: a lipreading
    screening test with implications for aural rehabili-
    tation, J. Speech Hearing Dis., 41, 530-539 (1976).

7. Birren, J. E. The Psychology of Aging. Englewood
    Cliffs, N.J.: Prentice-Hall (1964).

8. Botwinick, J. Aging and Behavior, New York: Springer
    (1973).

9. Cowdry, E. V. Problems of Aging, Baltimore: The
    Williams and Wilkins Co. (1939).

10. Donahue, W. Psychologic Aspects. Chapter in Cowdry,
    E. V. and Steinberg, F. U. (Eds.) The Care of the
    Geriatric Patient. St. Louis: The C. V. Mosby
    Co. (1971).

11. Dublin, E. B. Fundamentals of Neuropathology,
    Springfield, Ill.: Charles C. Thomas (1967).

12. Erber, N. P. Auditory, visual and auditory-visual
    recognition of consonants by children with normal
    and impaired hearing. J. Speech Hearing Res., 17,
    413-422 (1972).

13. Erber, N. P. Effects of angle, distance and illumina-
    tion on visual reception of speech by profoundly
    deaf children. J. Speech Hearing Res., 17, 99-112
    (1974).

14. Erber, N. P. Interaction of audition and vision in
    the recognition of speech material. J. Speech
    Hearing Res., 12, 423-425 (1969).

15. Ewertsen, H. W. and Nielsen, H. Birk. A comparative
    analysis of the audiovisual, auditive and visual
    perception of speech. Acta Otolaryng., 72,
    201-205 (1971).

16. Farrimond, T. Age differences in the ability to use visual cues in auditory communication. *Lang. Speech,* *2,* 179-192 (1959).

17. Goetzinger, C. P. A study of monocular versus binocular vision in lipreading. Proceedings of the International Congress of Education of the Deaf and 41st Meeting of the Convention of American Instructors of the Deaf. Washington, D.C.: U.S. Government Printing Office, 326-333 (1963).

18. Hardick, E. J., Oyer, H. J. and Irion, P. E. Lipreading performance as related to measurements of vision. *J. Speech Hearing Res., 13,* 92-100 (1970).

19. Hood, R. B. and Dixon, R. F. Physical characteristics of speech rhythm of deaf and normal-hearing speakers. *J. Com. Dis., 2,* 20-28 (1969).

20. Kalish, R. A. The Later Years: Social Applications of Gerontology, Monterey, California: Brooks/Cole Publishing Co. (1977).

21. Lovering, L. J. and Hardick, E. J. Lipreading performance as a function of visual acuity. Paper presented at the Annual Meeting of the American Speech and Hearing Association, Chicago, Ill. (1969).

22. Metropolitan Life Insurance Company. Hearing Impairments in the United States. Metropolitan Life Insurance Statistics, 57, 7-9 (1976).

23. Pelson, R. O. and Prather, W. F. Effects of visual message-related cues, age and hearing impairment on speechreading performance. *J. Speech Hearing Res., 17,* 518-525 (1974).

24. Pitorak, E. F. Diseases of the eye. Chapter in Moidel, H. C., Sorensen, G. E., Giblin, E. C. and Kaufman, M. A. Nursing care of the patient with medical-surgical disorders. New York: McGraw-Hill Book Co. (1971).

25. Riegel, K. A study of verbal achievement of older persons. *Journal of Gerontology, 14,* 453-456 (1956).

26.   Sanders, D. A. Aural Rehabilitation, Englewood Cliffs,
        N.J.: Prentice-Hall, Inc. (1971).

27.   Sanders, T. E. and Smith, M. E. Opthalmic Aspects.
        Chapter in Cowdry, E. V. and Steinberg, F. U. (Eds.)
        The Care of the Geriatric Patient. St. Louis:
        The C. V. Mosby Co. (1971).

28.   Schow, R. L., Christensen, J. M., Hutchinson, J. M. and
        Nerbonne, M. A. Communication Disorders of the Aged,
        Baltimore: University Park Press (1978).

29.   Schuknecht, H. Further observations on the pathology
        of presbycusis. *Archives of Otolaryngology, 80,*
        369-382.

30.   Shoop, C. and Binnie, C. A. The effect of age on the
        visual perception of speech. *Scandinavian Audiology,*
        7, (1978).

31.   U.S. Department of Health, Education and Welfare.
        Cataract and Glaucoma, Public Health Service Publica-
        tion No. 793, Health Information Series No. 99.
        Washington, D.C.: Government Printing Office (1963).

32.   Wallace, J. Some studies of perception in relation to
        age. *British Journal of Psychology, 47,* 283-297
        (1956).

33.   Weale, R. A. On the eye. In A. T. Welford and J. E.
        Birren (Eds.), Behavior, Aging and the Nervous
        System. Springfield, Ill.: Charles C. Thomas (1965).

34.   Weiss, A. D. Sensory functions. Chapter in Birren,
        J. E. (Ed.), Handbook of Aging and the Individual:
        Psychological and Biological Aspects. Chicago:
        University of Chicago Press (1959).

DISCUSSION

Audience: Some older people require more time to
respond; to repeat verbally to something that they have
heard. Dr. Binnie, were any of these tests modified to allow
for that?

Binnie: They were modified to the point that ample
time was provided to all subjects. I do not think that I
mentioned during the presentation of the paper that the
response time was a "write down" procedure. There were prepared answer sheets. We started the videotape system, presented the stimulus, put the videotape on pause while individuals responded by writing.

Audience: Did the subjects commit the error of
omission which a lot of people talk about? Was it a forced
response?

Binnie: The answer is yes and no. It depends basically upon the stimulus material. The CV syllable format
was a closed response. There were 20 orthographic symbols
representing the 20 consonants and the individuals were required to give a response because even if they guessed, it
could be that the scores would fall within one of the consonant clusters. They left the sentence blank in many cases.

Audience: Were there a lot of "no" responses during
the sentence stimuli?

Binnie: I cannot remember in terms of the item
analysis. It was very hard to motivate them to give complete
answers. They put down whatever they thought they saw. Many
times it was a phrase, but it was not complete. That was one
thing that we encouraged. If they had any idea what it might
be, we wanted them to go ahead and write a word or three and
try to make a sentence out of it.

Cooper: If I heard correctly, you said there were
increasing omissions with age so that the younger people put
down more words. Did the older people put down fewer words
with more blanks?

Binnie: I did not do that close of an analysis.

Cooper: Is that your gut feeling at this stage?

Binnie: Yes.

Audience: I am concerned about the people who appear
not to be able to use visual cues to increase their speech
discrimination ability. Dr. Garstecki, with your subjects
that did not show improvement, did you use evoked response
or any other types of central testing to see if there was
some measureable process difference that would allow for
prediction about those people who can profit from contextual

cue training? Also, did you use visual cues only, and
visual plus auditory cues and then auditory cues alone?
I have tested some people who showed no improvement with
speechreading with audition as opposed to speechreading with
visual cues alone. I was wondering if you could tell me
about that?

   Garstecki: We did not do any further evaluation of our subjects. My observation of their everyday performance was that they avoided interpersonal communication.
They were the "loner" type. It would be interesting to see
if we could find physiological data to support this apparent
lack of ability to use all available situational cue information. I think this would be the next step.

   For the situational cue task we did present the
material in the visual only mode, although that certainly
is another step, it would seem to have limited prescriptive
value. Unfortunately, I have not been able to collect running data from the same subject groups.

Chapter 9

Some Characteristics of Temporal
Auditory Behavior Among
Elderly Persons

ROBERT L. MC CROSKEY, PH. D.

I recognize that it is customary to begin with the
development of the rationale and the background to an investigation and then report the procedure and the results, but in
this instance it seems more reasonable to provide the results
first and then talk about why those results may have been obtained, and finally discuss the rehabilitation implications.

About twenty years ago I began talking about the concept of an *Auditory Age*. At that time I was concerned with
hearing impaired infants. I described the three-year-old
hearing impaired child, who had never had amplification, as a
geriatric case with respect to the development of speech and
language. The notion was that if a child had lived for several years with inadequate hearing available to him, his
chronological age would not match his auditory experiential
age and, in fact, at the time that amplification became available he must be considered an auditory newborn. (This seemed
to help parents understand that there must be approximately
a 12-month period of auditory stimulation, beginning at
Auditory Age zero, before they should expect that baby to begin to produce words.)

In the last five years, the application of the concept
of Auditory Age to the aging adult has begun to take form.
Since physiologic maturation and acoustic experience influence
the type and quality of response of very young listeners
(McCroskey, 1967; McCroskey and Herman, 1971), it is reasonable to project reverse effects stemming from degenerative
effects. The possible roles of regressive anatomic and physiologic components among the elderly, plus some decrement in
auditory experience as a function of increasing hearing impairment, has been explored and some of these contributions
will be discussed in a later section.

One critical element in the determining of the integrity of an auditory system is temporal discrimination. Consider first the definitions of two procedures--auditory fusion

and auditory processing--that have been used to look at temporal integrity. Auditory fusion has been viewed in a
variety of ways, but for the purposes of this report auditory
fusion is defined as the duration of a silent interval between two brief tone-bursts that is just-not-noticeable by a
listener. In other words, it is the point at which two tone-
bursts are so close together that the listener perceives them
as a single event. Thus, the finer the resolution characteristics of the auditory system, the better the detection of
silent intervals between tone-bursts.

Data have now been collected on approximately 700 individuals between three years of age and 70 years of age.
For centuries, artists, poets and philosophers have described
the seven ages of man, and all depict the similarity between
the two ends of the age spectrum. Let us consider the performance of the younger listeners first. At three years of
age the silent interval between two, 17-millisecond (msec)
tone-bursts is just-not-noticeable for normal children when
the silent interval is approximately 23 msec in duration.

Temporal resolution appears to improve dramatically
from three years of age to nine years of age, at which time
fusion occurs at approximately six milliseconds. There is an
interesting relationship between age and auditory temporal
proficiency. If one considers the ages of three, six, nine,
and twelve years, it may be noted that for each 3-year age
increment the auditory fusion point is approximately halved.
Earlier work by McCroskey and Cory (1968), revealed the same
pattern for temporal ordering. In that work, the interpulse
interval was held constant while the durations of the members
of a pulse-pair were manipulated. The listener's task was to
report whether the short or the long tone came first. Their
results indicated that the duration of the tones of a pair
had to be different by at least 612 milliseconds for the
three-year old listeners, but with each three-year age increment, the threshold for temporal ordering descended to
approximately 300, 150, 75, and 35 msec (at age 15).

The relationship between duration discrimination for
tones and durational requirements in spoken communication may
be clarified by reflecting a moment on the usual rate at
which adults talk to very young children, to preschool children, to primary level children and so forth. An interesting
study was reported by Cuda and Nelson (1976) in which it was
shown that the rate of teachers' speech increased markedly
between the first and third grades, then remained stable
through the sixth grade; however, sentence length remained at
a fairly simple level through the third grade and did not increase markedly until sixth grade.

Now let us consider the relationship between the age of an individual and his auditory fusion point (AFP) as we move through several decades of life. Although no data have been collected on subjects from 12 through 19 years of age, it is possible to infer information from the data on 10- and 11-year-old listeners and data from 20-year-olds and older. At 11 years of age the fusion point is approximately 6 msec when all frequencies of tone-bursts are pooled, but when considering only the 1000 Hz tone, the fusion point is closer to five milliseconds at 11 years of age. By age 20, the fusion point has improved slightly to 4 milliseconds where it remains very stable through age 49; however, at age 50 there are indications that the fine-grain temporal resolution is beginning to diminish. By the sixth decade of life, the mean fusion point is similar to that of a six-year-old, except that the standard deviation is much greater for elderly individuals than it is for children. The fusion point for a six-year-old is approximately 13 milliseconds with a standard deviation of five while the fusion point for adults in their sixties is 11 milliseconds with a standard deviation of 14.

The data on auditory fusion of adults were collected on approximately 550 individuals attending a national professional meeting. It is possible that this sample may present a more optimistic picture than would be true for elderly people in general, since these listeners were professionally active and highly mobile. It is very likely that persons from more restrictive environments would show an earlier and more severe decrement in temporal resolution.

Before other data are presented and interpreted in the area of auditory fusion, it should be noted that the 20 subjects who participated in our most recent study (McCroskey and Schmitt, 1978) ranged in age from 65 to 88 years with a mean of 73.2 years. Their mean AFP was 23.6 msec--the equivalent of the AFP for three-year-old children. All listeners were active individuals who attended community centers for recreational and social purposes. To be eligible to participate, all individuals must have been in good health and have no history of ear pathology. It was not required that auditory thresholds be within normal limits. All stimuli were presented at a fixed intensity above each listener's threshold for the stimulus tones.

Each stimulus was composed of two, 17-millisecond tone-bursts separated by one of the following 15 discrete interburst intervals: 0, 2, 5, 10, 15, 20, 30, 40, 50, 60, 70, 80, 90 and 100 milliseconds. Response time was set at a constant 5-second duration. All stimuli were presented

binaurally through matched TDH-39 earphones that had no
interaural phase difference.

Stimulus intensities were established in terms of
Sensation Levels (SL) rather than direct decibel readings
from an audiometer. Sensation Level is measured in terms of
decibels above an individual's threshold; thus, it is possible to specify signal levels that are comparable for all
listeners, relative to their own thresholds. Fusion points
were obtained at intensity levels of 20, 40 and 60 dB SL in
the better ear for the 1000 Hz stimulus frequency. An arbitrary intensity of 50 dB SL was used for the 250 Hz and the
4000 Hz tones. This abbreviation of the procedure was an
attempt to avoid fatiguing of the listeners. It seemed justified in terms of the data available from an earlier study
indicating that auditory fusion does not change significantly
from 40 dB SL to 60 dB SL (McCroskey and Davis, 1976). The
50 dB intensity for the other two test frequencies was an
arbitrary decision to strike a midpoint.

Fusion points were approached in both ascending and
descending trials, according to a Method of Limits Procedure.
In the ascending trial, the interburst interval began at 0
milliseconds and proceeded to 100 milliseconds; in the descending trials, the interburst interval began at 100 milliseconds and proceeded to 0 milliseconds. A listener's task
was to record either a 1 or a 2 on a response form, depending
upon whether he perceived the stimulus as a single tone burst
or as a pair of sounds.

Normal young listeners perform basically the same regardless of the stimulus frequency. For these elderly listeners, the mean auditory fusion points (AFP) for the 250 Hz
and the 4000 Hz stimuli were significantly poorer than the
AFP for 1000 Hz (See Table 1).

Earlier data on normal, young ears indicates that
temporal discrimination improves with some increase in intensity, e.g., from 20 dB to 40 dB SL (McCroskey and Davis,
1976); however, this was not the case for the elderly listeners. In fact, they obtained poorer auditory fusion thresholds at 50 dB SL than at 20 dB SL (24 msec versus 23 msec).
The V-shaped pattern that characterized the auditory fusion
of the elderly (See Figure 1) is reminiscent of the configuration obtained for younger subjects (mean age = 7 years) who
had been diagnosed as learning disabled.

TABLE 1

A Summary of Analysis of Variance for five
selected frequency-intensity combinations
of the Wichita Auditory Fusion Test

SOURCE	SS	df	MS	F
Between				
Treatments	413.746	4	103.436	4.038**
Subjects	26344.609	19	1386.558	
Within (error)	1946.919	76	25.617	
Total	28705.274			

**Significant at .01 level

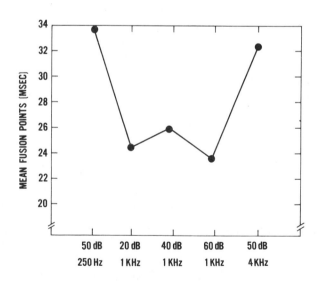

FIG. 1. The relative mean auditory fusion
points for elderly listeners according to
frequency (Hz) and intensity (dB SL) of
stimulus tone-pairs.

These listeners also show poorer fusion points for 250 Hz and
4000 Hz than they show at 1000 Hz. It is an interesting sim-
iliarity.

It must be noted that approximately 20% of the subjects exhibited auditory fusion points that were very similar
to those of young subjects while approximately 25% of the
elderly listeners yielded significantly higher fusion points.
This emphasizes the individuality of the aging individual and
possibly provides supportive evidence for the importance of
determining the Auditory Age of a listener.

The other major test procedure involved auditory processing of speech that had been subjected to electronic rate-
alteration. A number of researchers have reported that elderly listeners perform more poorly than young listeners on
speech discrimination tasks in which stimulus words have been
time-compressed (Bocca and Calearo, 1963; Sticht and Gray,
1969). Recently, Konkle, Beasley and Bess (1977) reported
that discrimination scores for time-compressed speech became
progressively worse from age 54 upward. Their data support
the results of the Wichita Auditory Fusion Test (McCroskey,
1975) with elderly listeners.

In view of the fact that it has been demonstrated
that rapid speech interferes with speech intelligibility, it
is surprising that there have not been more studies involving
slowed speech. Based on research with learning disability
(LD) children, McCroskey and Thompson (1973) found that a
modest slowing of speech rate facilitated comprehension by
young LD listeners. Given the fact that the auditory fusion
characteristics of the aged group are somewhat similar to the
fusion characteristics of the young LD group, it was hypothesized that expanded (slower-than-normal) speech would facilitate the comprehension of spoken sentences. McCroskey and
Schmitt (1978) presented four sets of 10 sentences that were
matched for length and linguistic complexity at four different rates of speaking. Rate alteration was accomplished with
an Eltro Information Rate Changer and recorded onto four
stimulus tapes.

One set of 10 sentences was processed at normal rate
(175 wpm); one was processed at a faster-than-normal rate
(291 wpm). The other two sets of sentences were processed at
two slower-than-normal rates (125 and 97 wpm). The subjects
heard the lists in random order. Four subjects were tested
simultaneously. All listening was under headphones (TDH-39).
The listener's task was to point to the correct picture from
among four choices. Each picture plate contained the correct
item plus three decoys. Each decoy contained either the

subject or the predicate, but only one sentence had the subject and predicate in the right combination.

The results of the analysis of variance indicated
that there were significant differences in sentence comprehension as a function of the rate at which sentences were
delivered (See Table 2).

TABLE 2

*Repeated Measures Analysis of Variance Source
Table for the four time-altered presentation
rates of the Wichita Auditory
Processing Test*

SOURCE	SS	df	MS	F
Between				
Treatments	1990	3	663.333	9.670**
Subjects	7780	19	409.474	
Within (error)	3910	57	68.596	
Total	13680	79		

**Significant at .01 level

Since there was a significant main effect, Scheffe post hoc
comparisons (Winer, 1971) were made among all pairs of means.
The results indicated that rate of speaking affects sentence
comprehension among elderly listeners, but not entirely in
the direction hypothesized. Electronic slowing of the speech
rate did, as expected, improve comprehension. Further, when
the degree of expansion exceeded certain limits (180%) there
was an adverse affect. This, like the data from the fusion
test, is quite similar to the pattern exhibited by LD children. One unexpected result was the improved speech comprehension that occurred under the compressed condition (291
wpm). These listeners did as well under the condition of
140% expansion as they did under the condition of 60%
compression.

There are several elements about this research that
need further study. The performance did not follow a consistent pattern with respect to rate, nor did the results agree
with some earlier studies that revealed poorer performance

under conditions of accelerated speech. It must be remembered, however, that these data were collected on whole sentences rather than word lists, as have been used previously.
Possible differential effects of types of stimuli are now
being researched by making direct comparisons of performance
under rate alteration of words, sentences and connected
discourse.

There is another element that may have contributed to
some of the unexpected results. These listeners were tested
in small groups and this may have created a competitive situation which resulted in improved attending to the task. The
possible effects of competitiveness cannot be extracted from
these data, nor can one do more than speculate upon the
attentional effects that may have contributed to improved
comprehension at both faster- and slower-than-normal rates
of speaking.

Given that auditory temporal integrity, as measured
by auditory fusion and rate altered speech, begins to change
as age advances, the question becomes one of how much does
it change and is it a shift that makes a difference. Is the
slowing of the timing function by 10-15 milliseconds a change
that could have impact on day-to-day performance? To answer
this question some attention must be given to the physical
parameters of speech itself.

RATIONALE

To state the obvious, speech is a complex activity.
Not only is it complicated in terms of psycho-neuromuscular
activity, as evidenced by its metabolic cost to a speaker
(McCroskey, 1957), but it is acoustically complex in terms of
the rapidly changing pattern that constitutes the speech act.
In spite of this complexity, the acoustic aspects of speech
can be analyzed in terms of just three physical parameters:
frequency, intensity, and time. One does not have to be an
expert to know that the most common procedure for determining
whether hearing is normal or not, is by measuring only two
dimensions of hearing--frequency and intensity. These *two*
parameters yield an audiogram from which inferences are drawn
that can mislead educators, physicians, audiologists, and
parents. If the audiogram is the basis for determining normalcy of hearing, and the audiogram is within normal limits,
then a hearing impairment is not considered to be a part of
the problem. *Time* is the forgotten aspect, to a large extent, both in testing and in aural rehabilitation procedures.

What *are* some of the time elements that contribute
to the interpreting of a speech signal? Consider the work

of Eimas, et al., (1971) in which babies one- and four-months
old were presented with CV (consonant-vowel) syllables that
differed only in the voice onset time (VOT) in initial consonants. Their work showed that VOTs that differed by approximately 20 msec were not only distinguishable but resulted in
behavioral differences. More recently, Lisker (1978) reported that a delay of 35 milliseconds (+ 15 msec) in the onset
of laryngeal vibration following release on an initial stop
consonant, generates acoustic features that elicit perceptions of /p, t, k/ from speakers of English. It is recognized, of course, that the time relationships for perceptions
of these kinds of phonemes differ from language to language--
which may be the explanation for an English speaking listener's perception of /b/ when a foreign speaker has actually
produced /p/. Lisker's work suggests that perception of some
speech events could require the detection of acoustic fea-
tures--and I include silence as an acoustic feature in speech
--as short as 20 milliseconds. Much of that type of research
has been accomplished using synthesized speech, but replica-
tion through the editing of natural speech, in order to control the duration of silent intervals corresponding to inter-
vocalic closure has been done, also (Port, 1976).

Speech is a time-ordered sequence of events that
makes accurate perception of temporal relationships critical
to comprehension. The fact that speech can be transcribed
using phonetic symbols may lead one to conclude that recognition and understanding will take place if one can hear a
string of phonemes that have common meaning among listeners
of a given group. Further reflection tells us that the meaning of these sequenced phonemes may be altered significantly
when a speaker alters the melody of the utterance or when the
speaker changes the stress pattern on some of the words.
Stress patterns are the product of intensity and time variations within an utterance. These factors involving pitch
variations and stress variations (prosody) are significant
to the comprehension of spoken verbal messages. Some work
using spectrograms of spontaneous speech reveal that syllables preceding judged-pause location were usually longer than
those following, whether or not a silent interval was present. Most judged-pause locations were junctures, but syllable length governed judgments independently of the juncture
cues (Martin, 1970). Martin's work suggests that individuals
generally detect 87% of pauses that are at least 50 msec in
duration, but silent intervals of less than 50 milliseconds
tend to be ignored as pauses. This should not be confused
with the fact that the pauses actually exist, as in a word
like "ladder" and, indeed, the silent interval that is

present is critical to the perception of the word. The relationship of timing patterns across phrases--as perceived by
listeners--may alter the reporting of a pause, and may influence listener identification of a pause, but it does not
negate the impact of the pause upon perception. Phrase-level
timing patterns as a function of stress have been studied by
Wisemer and Ingrisano (1978) and their data tend to support
the work of Lisker, inasmuch as it is not appropriate necessarily to assume that time programs for supraglottic struc-
tures dictate or are more important than time programs associated with laryngeal function. They hypothesize that the
reverse may be reasonable, especially if one views speech
production from the point of view than an independent rhythm
generator or internal clock exists and is sensitive to the
prosodic demands of an utterance rather than just the phono-
logical segment durations within the utterance.

It may be of interest to demonstrate some of the elements that contribute to perception. I will speak four words
to you and I would like you to write the four words that you
hear on a piece of paper. I will cover my mouth so that only
the acoustic information of the utterances will be available.
The words are: cat, cab, cap, and cad. Those who are familiar with phonetics will recognize that all of the words
ended with bilabial stop consonants. You may also realize
that in none of the four words was the final consonant re-
leased. Indeed, in one sense the final consonant was not
even spoken. Now, how accurately did you perform?[1] What was
heard that allowed the identification of the words? Each
sound of the English language has certain acoustic properties
and as one moves from one sound to the next there are some
frequency transitions that blend the two sounds together.
When one can perceive the direction of that blend, one can
predict the phoneme that is to come. Those who are familiar
with co-articulation or with progressive/regressive assimila-
tion, know that yet-to-be-spoken phonemes influence the production of phonemes that are in progress. Thus, in the words
that we just heard, there was a transition--a glide in the
frequency composition as one left the vowel sound of the word
and moved toward the final consonant. The perception of that
transition allowed you to predict the sound to come, even
when the sound was not heard. Think for a moment about the
sequence of movements through which your speech mechanism

---

[1]Listener accuracy was tallied and it was shown that there
was virtually 100% correct identification.

moves in order to progress through a word like "cat". One
can become aware that the mandible is more depressed for the
/æ/ than it is just before the final /t/ is to be approached.
To maintain predictibility a listener must be able to perceive these brief transitions. Here, one deals with a time
dimension of approximately 50 milliseconds.

As an illustration of the potential of pauses in
words to cause perception to take place as well as the effect of these transitions, we might listen to some pre-
programmed computer-generated speech as one might find in
the HandiVoice.[2] First, I will enter the four phonemes that
one would traditionally identify as composing the word
"nickel." Using the HandiVoice, I will enter each of the
phonemes of the word "nickel," following a phonetic tran-
scription model; then it will be entered with the /ə/ between the /k/ and the syllabic /l/; then the phonemes will
be entered in sequence except that a pause will be inserted
ahead of the /k/, as well as inserting the schwa sound between the k̲ and l̲; then, in the final production, the first
two phonemes and the syllabic l̲ will be entered and, instead
of the /k/, a *pause* will be inserted. The perception of the
word "nickel" is not significantly altered by the deletion
of the /k/ when it is replaced by a brief pause. Percep-
tually, listeners do hear and interpret the silent intervals.

Basically, it has been demonstrated that if the high
frequency components of a phoneme are not available to a
listener, either due to hearing loss or defective transducer,
the listener will perceive a phoneme other than the one that
was originally produced. The relationship of this information to temporal misinterpretation can be understood if one
reflects for a moment on the rise and fall characteristics
of sounds as they are initiated or terminated. For example,
as a speaker approaches the phoneme /b/ in the middle of a
word like "baby," there is a brief interval of silence, and,
as the speaker approaches that silent interlude there is
some period of time required for the sound of his voice to
reduce from its characteristic intensity to zero (the fall
time), and when the silent interval has been judged by the
speaker to have been appropriate, there is another period of
time required for the voice to increase from zero intensity

---

[2] HandiVoice is designed by the Vocal Interface Division of
the Federal Screw Works and is commercially available as
Phonic Mirror HandiVoice HC 110, H.C. Electronics, Inc.,
Mill Valley, California

to its characteristic intensity (the rise time). Persons
with normal hearing will detect the entire intensity range of
the fall/rise times, and will perceive the silent interval in
the same time frame in which the speaker produced it; however,
if there is a hearing impairment, the duration of the silent
interval will be perceived as being longer (See Figure 2).

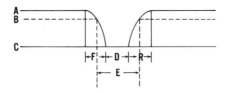

FIG. 2. A representation of the possible
effect of hearing loss on perceived duration
of interphonemic pause time (Line A is the
characteristic vocal intensity of one phoneme and Line C represents zero signal
intensity. The fall/rise times are shown
under the curved lines as durations F and
R. The real-time silent interval is D,
but the perceived silent interval is E
because of the hearing loss represented
by Line B).

This is accounted for by the fact that the full audible duration of signal decay and onset have been shortened by the
time/intensity portion that lies below a listener's threshold.
Since it can be demonstrated that the duration of the silent
interval results in different phonemic perceptions, and the
interaction of a hearing impairment with rise/fall times surrounding brief pauses in speech could influence the perception of the relative duration of that pause, it is hypothesized that there is another explanation for phonemic regression other than simple lack of availability of the higher
frequencies.

It is not difficult to find published reports showing
that aging listeners perform tasks at a slower rate. Hutchinson and Beasley (1976) refer to the reduction in the
speed of utterance among geriatric speakers. Based on their
observations, rather than specific data, they infer that maximum physiologic performance is reduced as a function of age.
Ryan (1972) also reports a progressive decrement in speaking
rate with increased age. His significance was obtained
between subjects in their fourth decade of life and subjects

in their seventh decade of life. The oldest group was significantly slower on tasks involving impromptu speaking and
oral reading. Speed of perception, speed of initiating a
response, and speed of movement are all involved in psycho-
motor performance. All three seem to be implicated in the
slowing that is seen as an accompaniment to advancing age or
to brain damage (Hicks and Birren, 1970). Extensive research
has been done on Response Time (RT) and there seems to be a
general feeling that the slower RTs are mainly centrally determined. This explanation is based partially on the belief
that velocity of signal conduction along the nerves is not
considered to alter significantly with advancing age (Wagman
and Lesse, 1952; Norris, Shock, and Wagman, 1953). It may
be important to note that Wagman and Lesse (1952) do not conclude that there is no change in neural velocity with aging,
but only that the magnitude of the decrement is judged to be
nonsignificant. Perhaps reappraisal of those results, in
light of the time requirements for the perception of acoustic
correlates in speech, would lead to reinterpretation of their
data.

The temporal relationship between sounds arriving at
Hearing impairment is generally accepted as a fact of
aging; notwithstanding the work of Powers and Powers (1978)
in which they suggest that a person who judges his hearing to
be very good at age 60 can anticipate continuing to enjoy
good hearing, and that the picture of the aged person as a
lonely individual with a hearing loss is an error. Whatever
reality is, the assumption exists that aging alone can account for the degenerative activity in the end organ of the
auditory system. The literature on the effect of aging upon
audition usually states that hair cells and supporting cells
are lost in the Organ of Corti as the result of aging
(Schucknecht, 1965). In view of the ubiquitous nature of
noise in today's environment, it is difficult to distinguish
pathological changes in the cochlea that may have resulted
from aging, from those changes that may be the result of
noise exposure. Regardless of the cause, atrophy can be
documented in the basal turn of the cochlea and this results
in high-frequency hearing impairment. According to Eldridge
(1974), the high-frequency portion of the basilar membrane
may also serve to preserve fine-grain temporal order of
acoustic events.

The temporal relationship between sounds arriving at
the two ears of a listener is known to contribute to localization of sound. Impaired localization has been associated
with presbycusis (Hinchcliffe, 1962). Much attention has
been given to changes within the inner ear but very little
attention has been given to the possible effects of the

documented changes that occur in the external ear. Not all
external ears change in the same way. For example, Zucker
and Williams (1977) describe the lengthening and the change
in resiliency of cartilages that support the external ear.
At the same time, there are descriptions of increased rigidity
of the pinna and an increase in the size of the external canal
(Schow, et al., 1978). However, most of the audiology books
contend that this appendage on the head contributes very
little if anything to the hearing process. Batteau (1964)
challenged that concept and suggested that the configuration
of the pinna contributed to the ability of a listeners to
localize sound in space. The phenomenon is easily illustra-
ted by simply bending the pinna into an unfamiliar shape; for
example, folding the superior aspect outward and downward in
order to form approximately a right angle with the long, ver-
tical axis of the pinna. Under these conditions, localization of a complex signal is very difficult. The hypothesis
is that the configuration of the external ear splits a complex signal into components that are delivered at slightly
different time intervals. These relative temporal relationships permit rather precise localization. Again, one may
conclude that anything that interferes with temporal relationships will contribute to distortion of that acoustic event.

    Some researchers have attempted to study the effect
of temporal distortion by delaying auditory feedback (Black,
1951; Lee, 1951) and by eliminating tactile feedback
(McCroskey, 1956). McCroskey's data showed that the effects
of disrupted tactile cues were very similar to the effects
of delayed auditory side-tone--both resulted in a slowing of
speech production. One may infer that anything that disrupts
the normal perception of time, whether it is by touch or by
ongoing auditory monitoring, results in an alteration of
speech rate. Inversely, slowed speech may reflect changes
that have taken place in the auditory, tactile and kinesthetic feedback systems.

    Auditory Age, as a concept, appears to be supported
by the research that has been labeled as the verbal transformation effect (Warren, 1961; Warren and Warren, 1966, 1970).
The verbal transformation effect refers to the phenomenon
whereby a listener perceives changes in a single, clearly
pronounced verbal stimulus that is repeated at a fixed repetition rate over a period of a few minutes. The Warren data
indicate that young people under five years of age do not experience such transformations, nor do individuals who are over
60 years of age. These data may be related significantly to
the results of the tests dealing with rate altered sentences.
In that experiment, the elderly listeners performed better

when the speech rate was made faster or slower than normal.
It may be that some of the same underlying mechanisms that
account for the lack of verbal transformations also account
for the improvement that occurs with changing rates of
speaking.

IMPLICATIONS FOR REHABILITATION

The goal of this paper has been to familiarize you
with the significance of time and timing in the reception
and understanding of spoken communication, so that you could
decide whether rehabilitation would be enhanced if certain
adjustments were to be made in spoken interchanges between
rehabilitationists and clients, and between clients and their
families.

In summary, it has been shown: (a) that each person
has an *Auditory Age* which may or may not match chronological
age, (b) that physical changes in the external, middle, and
inner ear contribute to inefficient temporal functions, (c)
that age is related to the efficiency with which an auditory
system can detect critical durational values in on-going
speech, (d) that small durational differences of both sound
and silence can alter recognition/perception of a spoken
event, (e) that rate-altered speech affects comprehension of
spoken sentences in a way that is different from comprehension of spoken single words, and (f) that the responses of
elderly listeners to tones and speech are similar to those
exhibited by learning disability children.

Effective rehabilitation relies on good communication. The information presented here clearly shows that communication will be improved if there is awareness of the need
for slower-than-normal rate of speaking with elderly
listeners.

It is a major importance that both the elderly and
their families be aware that some of the confusion and misunderstanding that arises is a function of a slowing auditory
system--an advancing auditory age--and not necessarily a di-
minuation of intellect. Further, when messages are delivered
at a comprehensible rate, the full import of the communication is more likely to be retained.

To know that communication is improved if the message
is spoken more slowly, and to be able to do it are two different things. Speech patterns are strongly ingrained and it
is only with some practice that a person can slow the delivery rate. The rehabilitation worker must practice the adage
"Make haste slowly." In the midst of pressure to get many
things done, it becomes important to give the impression of a

leisurely pace--by manner and by rate of talking. Perhaps
the most significant aspect of the kind of research reported
here is the potential for improving the level of respect between the aged and their families, and within the aged person, himself. It is important to have a reason for the difficulty experienced in understanding spoken communication.
It is important to know that some individuals may be understood less well because of the rate at which they talk and
not because the listener is no longer capable of understanding speech. The respect given and the respect felt could be
improved with the understanding of the role of time in spoken
communication.

REFERENCES

1. Batteau, D. W. Auditory perception. Final report,
    contract N123-(60540) 35401A, U.S. Naval Ordinance
    Test Station, China Lake, California, 1964.

2. Black, J. W. The effect of delayed side-tone upon vocal
    rate and intensity. *Journal of Speech and Hearing
    Disorders, 16,* 1951, 56-60.

3. Bocca, E. and Calearo, C. Central hearing processes.
    In Jerger, J. (Ed.), Modern Developments in Audiology.
    Academic Press, Inc., New York, 1963, 337-370.

4. Cuda, R. and Nelson, N. W. Analysis of speaking rate,
    syntactic complexity and speaking style of public
    school teachers. A paper presented to the National
    Convention of the American Speech and Hearing Associa-
    tion, Houston, Texas, 1976.

5. Eimas, P. D., Siqueland, E. R., Jusczyk, P., and
    Vigorito, J. Speech perception in infants. *Science,
    171,* 1971, 303-306.

6. Eldredge, D. H. Inner ear--Cochlear mechanics and coch-
    lear potentials. In Artrum, H., Jung, R., Loewen-
    stein, W. R., McKay, D. M., Teuber, H. L., (Eds.),
    Handbook of Sensory Physiology. Springer-Verlag
    Publishers, Berlin, 1974.

7. Hicks, L. H. and Birren, J. E. Aging, brain damage, and
    psychomotor slowing. *Psychological Bulletin, 74,*
    1970, 377-396.

8. Hinchcliffe, R. The anatomical locus of presbycusis.
    Journal of Speech and Hearing Disorders, 27, 1962,
    301-310.

9. Hutchinson, J. M. and Beasley, D. S. Speech and lang-
    uage functioning among the aging. In Oyer and Oyer
    (Eds.), <u>Aging and Communication.</u> University Park
    Press, Baltimore, 1976, p. 164.

10. Konkle, D. F., Beasley, D. S., and Bess, F. H. Intelli-
    gibility of time-altered speech in relation to chron-
    ological aging. *Journal of Speech and Hearing
    Research, 20,* 1977, 108-115.

11. Lee, B. S. Artificial stutterer. *Journal of Speech and
    Hearing Disorders, 16,* 1951, 53-55.

12. Lisker, L. Closure Hiatus: Cue to voicing, manner and
    place of consonant occlusion. <u>HASKINS LABORATORIES:
    Status Report on Speech Research SR-53,</u> 1978, 79-86.

13. Martin, J. G. On judging pauses in spontaneous speech.
    Journal of Verbal Learning and Verbal Behavior, 9,
    1970, 75-78.

14. McCroskey, R. L. Some effects of anesthetizing the
    articulators under conditions of normal and delayed
    side-tone. Research Report #65, Sub-Task I: The
    Ohio State University Research Foundation and U.S.
    School of Aviation Medicine, Pensacola, Florida,
    1956.

15. McCroskey, R. L. The effect of speech upon metabolism:
    A comparison between stutterers and non-stutterers.
    Journal of Speech and Hearing Disorders, 22, 1957,
    46-52.

16. McCroskey, R. L. A new device for screening neonates.
    A paper presented to the National Convention of the
    American Speech and Hearing Association, Chicago,
    1967.

17. McCroskey, R. L. <u>Wichita Auditory Fusion Test.</u> Depart-
    ment of Logopedics, Wichita State University, Wichita
    Kansas, 1975.

18. McCroskey, R. L. and Cory, M. Duration discrimination
     by children from three to 16 years of age. A paper
     presented to the National Convention of the American
     Speech and Hearing Association, Denver, 1968.

19. McCroskey, R. L. and Davis, S. M. Auditory fusion--
     Developmental trends. A scientific exhibit presented
     to the National Convention of the American Speech and
     Hearing Association, Houston, Texas, 1976.

20. McCroskey, R. L. and Herman, N. Some effects of certain
     auditory experiences upon responsiveness of human
     neonates. *Journal of Kansas Speech and Hearing
     Association*, 1971, 68-76.

21. McCroskey, R. L. and McCroskey, J. B. Some effects of
     speaking rate and intensity upon verbal transforma-
     tions. An unpublished manuscript, 1975.

22. McCroskey, R. L. and Schmitt, J. F. Auditory temporal
     processing among elderly adults. Unpublished re-
     search paper. Wichita State University, Grant
     #3399-22, Wichita, Kansas, 1978.

23. McCroskey, R. L. and Thompson, N. W. Comprehension of
     rate-controlled speech by children with specific
     learning disabilities. *Journal of Learning Disabili-
     ties, 6,* 1973, 621-627.

24. Norris, A. H., Shock, N., and Wagman, I. Age changes in
     the maximum conduction velocity of motor fibers of
     human ulnar nerves. *Journal of Applied Physiology,
     5,* 1953, 589-593.

25. Port, R. The influence of tempo on the closure interval
     cue to the voicing and place of intervocalic stops.
     Journal of the Acoustical Society of America, 59,
     Supplement 1, 1976, S41-42.

26. Powers, J. K. and Powers, E. A. Hearing problems of
     elderly persons: Social consequences and prevalence.
     ASHA, 20, 1978, 79-83.

27. Ryan, W. J. Acoustic aspects of the aging voice.
     Journal of Gerontology, 27, 1972, 165-168.

28. Schow, R. L., Christensen, J. M., Hutchinson, J. M. and
     Nerbonne, M. A. Communication Disorders of the Aged.
     University Park Press, Baltimore, 1978.

29. Schucknecht, H. F. The effect of aging on the cochlea.
     Proceedings of International Symposium on Sensori-
     neural Hearing Processes and Disorders. Little,
     Brown and Company, Boston, 1965, 393-401.

30. Sticht, T. and Gray, B. The intelligibility of time-
     compressed words as a function of age and hearing
     loss. Journal of Speech and Hearing Research, 12,
     1969, 443-448.

31. Wagman, I. H. and Lesse, H. Maximum conduction veloci-
     ties of motor fibers of ulnar nerve in human sub-
     jects of various ages and sizes. Journal of Neuro-
     physiology, 15, 1952, 235-244.

32. Warren, R. M. Illusory changes in repeated words:
     differences between young adults and the aged.
     American Journal of Psychology, 52, 1961, 249-258.

33. Warren, R. M. and Warren, R. P. A comparison of speech
     perception in childhood, maturity, and old age by
     means of the verbal transformation effect. Journal
     of Verbal Learning and Verbal Behavior, 5, 1966,
     142-146.

34. Warren, R. M. and Warren, R. P. Auditory illusions and
     confusions. Scientific American, 223, 1970, 30-36.

35. Weismer, G. and Ingrisano, D. R. Phrase-level timing
     patterns and precision as a function of emphatic-
     stress location within an utterance. Accepted for
     publication in Journal of Speech and Hearing
     Research, 1978.

36. Winer, B. J. Statistical principles in experimental
     design. McGraw-Hill, New York, 1971.

37. Zucker, K., and Williams, P. Audiological services in
     an extended care facility. Paper presented at
     Annual Convention of the American Speech and Hearing ·
     Association, Chicago, 1977.

Chapter 10

Psychological and Social Aspects
of Aging as Related to Hearing
Rehabilitation of Elderly Clients

JEROME G. ALPINER, PH. D.

Contemporary society has made numerous judgments regarding the phenomenon of aging, not simply because we wanted to say someone was growing older but rather because a definition of the process was apparently needed. Little did we realize that definitions would linger and cast negative connotations in an era in which commitments emerged regarding rehabilitation of persons with handicapping conditions; for the audiologist the commitment was for improvement of communication function for persons with hearing loss. During the past two decades, rehabilitation for the older American became an increased concern for many professional individuals in a variety of disciplines.

We have become aware of the physiological problems resulting from the aging process. There are more than 12 million senior citizens who have certain chronic conditions such as heart disease, arthritis, diabetes and mental disorders among the more than 20 million persons past the age of 65 (U.S. Senate Special Committee on Aging, 1971). These conditions cause constant discomfort and limit the activities of many persons. Further, we realize that the older American has decreased income for sustenance, many hours of leisure time since regularity of work no longer exists, and fewer friends with whom to associate due to the fact that mobility becomes more difficult and former friends are deceased. It is appropriate for audiologists to advocate utilization of amplification and rehabilitation procedures. Not to do so would imply that we believe our procedures are inadequate and little hope exists for assisting the older American. We need to admit, however, that this population is not quite the same as groups of children or middle age adults, for example, who presumably have a productive future. Yet, there are those of us who will contend that all years of life should be meaningful and that we should plan remediation appropriately. At the present time there is no fully

accepted psychology of aging as related to hearing loss.
There are trends, however, which will be discussed in terms
of an emerging psycho-social pattern for older Americans.
There first is a need to overcome the barriers of definition
that have plagued this population for many years. These
barriers are not necessarily direct obstacles for audiologists in the sense that what we do is not meaningful but
rather the meaning they have for persons for whom we provide
service. What are these negative connotations possessed by
so many persons in the United States? A semantic perspective
indicates that the elderly are older, more mature, and aged.
Attempts to substitute the term with elderly results in somewhat of a vicious circle since aged happens to be one of the
definitions of elderly. The antonym of both elderly and
aged is youth - a reminder to the older individual that
being young is something now past.

From a medical point of view, older persons are referred to in contexts of gerontology and geriatrics; gerontology is the study of "old" age and geriatrics is the study
and treatment of the diseases of "old" age. The topic of
this paper deals with psychological and social aspects of
aging as related to hearing rehabilitation of elderly clients. Social means friendly and interdependent. Psychology
refers to a science which deals with the mind, its functions,
its powers and its acts. The word rehabilitation implies a
restoration to a former condition or to put in good condition again. Defined in specific context, its meaning implies that we will restore a person, in this case a person
with various physiological problems to a former condition
which tended toward normalcy. Theoretically, rehabilitation
is appropriate. How, then, can we convey this concept of
Rehabilitation to those older individuals who have been defined as less than perfect by physicians, other persons, and
semantics? Is it possible that we have created nomenclature
that is self-destructing in terms of concepts and attitudes
which label the person age 65 and over as old, and the person
believes that he is old and incapable of remediation.

If large numbers of older Americans indeed feel that
they are at terminal stages in their lives, if they believe
that society has relegated them to "have beens", the hearing
aids, counseling, and rehabilitative audiology are of no
import in everyday living. After all, one out of every four
persons age 65 and over lives in poverty compared to one out
of nine who are younger (U.S. Senate Committee on Aging,
1971). Changing health care provisions make adequate protection doubtful with regard to such aspects as prescription
drugs, eyeglasses, dentures, and hearing aids (Kimmel, 1974).

And if we are concerned about psychology and the function of
the mind, you probably will recall the numerous media adver-
tisements that stress a discount for the senior citizen because that person is "old". Housing generally is inadequate
due to reduced income and many of these persons do not live
where they wish. In most areas of the United States, conven-
ient transportation is not available and older Americans are
not able to go where they want to, when they want to.
Another significant problem which sets apart these individuals is nutrition. This situation was well stated by Muskie
(1971) who said, "dry economic statistics can never convey
the emotional meaning of growing old in poverty, often in
dangerous urban neighborhoods, and of having to choose between money for food or money for desperately needed medical
care."

If we are willing to accept the general information
regarding aging as well as the fact that between 30 and 90%
of this population have significant hearing impairment (U.S.
Senate Committee on Aging, 1968; Chaffee, 1967, Hull and
Traynor, 1977), a dilemma confronts us. What is the most
important situation confronting the older American: health,
transportation, housing, nutrition, hearing problems, being
old? Perhaps, more important, how do all of these factors
inter-relate for the overall welfare of the individual? Let
us exclude those persons who are physically and/or mentally
unable to assume any responsibilities for everyday living.
We still have the situations previously mentioned. The physician may say that the general health condition is the most
important, and the audiologist may say that hearing is the
most important. The senior citizen may say, "I don't care,
I am old and it is too difficult to cope with the demands of
society". The contention of this contributor is that all
factors are important but that the most important consideration is the need to create a psychological attitude that
negates the hopelessness of feeling old.

Alpiner (1964) found that older Americans in "homes
for the aged" and in a self sustaining retirement center
possessed three major attitudes regarding hearing rehabilitation: (1) a definite denial that a hearing problem was
present, (2) an attitude of hopelessness regarding life; i.e.
time should be spent with younger persons who would live
longer, and (3) a recognition of hearing loss but no desire
for hearing rehabilitation. These were psychological attitudes and a generalization was unfortunately made that all
older persons felt this way. After 14 years of working in
hearing rehabilitation with so called senior citizens
(approximately 3,000 persons), this author realized that

numerous factors had to be considered and that one could not
generalize to the three attitudes initially indicated. This
position change emerged as a result of studies investigating
hearing impaired individuals through communication function
assessment inventories which compared persons with themselves rather than with groups of persons. In reality, the
philosophy was one of coping with persons on an individual
basis regardless of age. It was a matter of dealing with
people and their unique psychology. There were older persons
who functioned like everyone else, even though concomitant
problems such as health constraints existed. Their pre-
morbid personalities dictated that they would lead a life
style that was geared to communication. These individuals
were easy to work with in therapy; they were committed to
making life worthwhile in spite of physical, economic, and
society difficulties. Their motivation to be self sustaining was enhanced by the audiologist who provided them with
amplification and rehabilitative therapy. These people were
involved in a remediation process that was not much different than those adults below the age of 65. That is not to
say that problems were not encountered but rather to say
that the element of "hopeless" old age was not involved in
the remediation process. They accepted the "routine" procedures of audiologic assessment, hearing aid evaluation,
and remediation therapy.

       An attempt then was made to ascertain the contribu-
ting factors, if any, to a psychology of aging as related to
hearing loss. It appeared not to be so simple a situation
as related only to hearing loss. Mead (1962) suggested that
prevention might possibly be the best way to approach the
psychological problems which manifest themselves in so many
older adults. The significance of Mead's work was that individuals should be prepared for growing older in a positive
manner. In essence, what are the advantages afforded by the
later years? This approach is different than what previously
has been described as the "psychological dilemma" of being
old. It even necessitates a change in the semantics of des-
cribing persons in their sixties, seventies, etc. It means
that we do away with the television commercials, in their
present format that imply that this population should drink
decaffeinated coffee, or use a certain denture glue, or take
iron as a supplement to keep up with younger persons. If we
are not able to really be willing to change our own attitudes, then Mead may be quite correct in what behavioral
characteristics might emerge:

1. <u>Turning to childish superficial satisfactions</u>. This type of reaction may exist because the older person cannot look ahead to the future. A number of clients attempt to evade focusing on therapy by telling jokes about their childhood. This is not a bad situation but if the entire focus of the therapy session is in this direction, it is doubtful if progress in communication function may be achieved. Related to this mechanism is the situation in which clinicians continually treat adults like children: Hello, honey, how is the girl today? Don't be sad, you will do better next time. The childish vocal intonations accompanying these types of statements are those we might use with young children in therapy.

2. <u>Denial mechanism</u>. This client is the one who denies old age by resorting to such things as health fads. There are those clients who insist that certain vitamins will reverse a hearing loss or make their vision better. They may state that hearing loss is not due to aging but rather a deficiency in diet by not eating the appropriate foods.

3. <u>Non-acceptance of the aging process</u>. This person is one who does not accept the idea that the disability is caused by aging. Other reasons are sought for the cause of the disorder. We have encountered clients who state, for example, that hearing loss was caused by a serious accident to the head during childhood or that they had an illness for which the cause was unknown. The outright refusal to consider the aging process as a possible cause of the problem seems to be the pattern for this particular category.

4. <u>Inability to accept the changes of old age</u>. This person is relegated to a state of depression or apathy. This is not due solely to the hearing loss but is seen as only one traumatic aspect of the multitude of disorders which may accompany aging such as heart disease and diabetes.

5. <u>Senility</u>. The final reaction may result from actual cortical deterioration resulting in senility. This condition precludes the audiologist from engaging in therapy. A caution must be inserted in this category. We have encountered clients who appear to be senile but actually possess severe discrimination problems. They are labeled senile falsely and Alpiner refers to this particular situation as "pseudo senility." The situation most often has been encountered in extended care facilities in which staffs have not been appropriately trained regarding the manifestations of hearing impairment.

To the previously mentioned emotional and social problems of aging, which may set certain older persons apart from the mainstream of everyday living, the handicap of hearing loss may be added as a real entity. We tend to associate aging with presbycusis. Presbycusic ramifications have been viewed in terms of increased withdrawal and isolation, increased insecurity, and emotional stress. Hearing loss, therefore, can be a significant factor in the aging process, increasing dependence and the need for assistance (Myklebust, 1968). It may be helpful to reverse the process and view the person who is born deaf or acquires hearing impairment at an early age (Wolff, 1959). There is no more important factor in the emotional adjustment of hearing loss than isolation. There is a deficient monitoring system which affects one's thoughts and feelings. We know that when a normal hearing person is deprived of sensory stimulation, he becomes disturbed because the means to monitor feelings and ideas are distorted. To add to the feeling of isolation is the fact that the hearing impaired person may be regarded as somewhat a part of a minority group. Normal hearing individuals shy away from old "senile" persons. It is easier to avoid these persons than to communicate with them.

Not all older citizens, as previously mentioned, undergo the social and emotional problems discussed. Some, as a matter of fact, find old age fun and challenging. Why? It helps to have good health and money to spend, but the key seems to be to stay active and participate in one's community. Get a job; join in the movement to support the rights and needs of older persons. The older individual should be helped, when necessary, to take part in community activity. Leadership roles should be encouraged. Employment of some type should be sought. Sports, crafts, and other talents should be rediscovered or assumed. There are church groups, bridge groups, fund raising groups, discussion groups, garden clubs. The list of organizations is endless in which older individuals can become involved. The danger is that in limiting themselves to senior citizens alone, these programs could be responsible for creating a subculture. Our goal should be to keep them integrated and productive rather than to see how successfully we can turn them over to the care of the organized, exclusive senior clubs and residences. There must be, therefore, a facilitator who keeps these individuals involved whether or not they live in an extended care facility or in a private residence. Is the facilitator to be an audiologist, a psychologist, a social worker, or someone else? There is no clear answer to this question at this point in time. The important consideration is that these

may develop a frame of mind that keeps senior citizens in the
mainstream, individuals who may otherwise withdraw. There is
no easy solution; otherwise the problem situation of who the
facilitator is to be would already have been resolved. From
the communication viewpoint, the audiologist may be a facilitator with regard to how the individual views himself. It
would be a positive situation, however, if the client was
able to engage in productive community activity once the
hearing therapy session was over for the day or week. Have
you ever wondered what that client was doing during the
course of the week after therapy was finished? Have you ever
encountered the feeling: "Has it really been worthwhile,
what have I accomplished?" At this point, we must now keep
in mind that we are addressing ourselves to the individual
client; what are his needs, how we may best assess them, and
what is the appropriate course of action for remediation. We
may then begin to develop an individual profile of the older
person, a psychology, so-to-speak, of attitudes toward the
environment.

A prerequisite exists to the above. This writer believes that we must do away with present nomenclature regarding old age. The task will not be easy to accomplish since
we are dealing with tradition, we are contending with an
attitude that has existed for many years. The task is a
challenge since it always is difficult to change a way of
thinking, a process that has been comfortable, even though
not practical, to live with. It is proposed that the terminology that designates an age group; i.e. older American, the
elderly, the aged, the mature, etc. be changed. It is rec-
commended that reference be made to adults and only to adults
without a preceding adjective. The audiologist cannot accomplish this mission alone since we address ourselves to the
way all persons view the process of "growing". We may not be
ready for this stage of growth but the attempt must be made.
As there are individual differences with children, there are
differences with adults. As there are mechanisms with which
parents deal with hearing impaired children, so must there be
differences with the way family members deal with their relatives, whatever the relationship. As we have advocated
rights for all individuals, let us advocate this same philosophy for all adults.

If we agree to this assumption, then the psychology
of the supposed aging process is not based on age but rather
is based on relationships that exist within the environment.
What is frustrating to this author at this point is the nomenclature which makes reference to age, at least at this
point in time. It indeed is difficult to deviate from the

traditional point of view. From a psychological point of
view, regarding the role of the audiologist, the characteristics for study of relationships between adults emerge from
the following categories: family, emotional, other persons,
general communication, self concepts, group situations, and
rehabilitation. When the term senior citizen emerges, it is
because there is no other appropriate way to refer to the
individual. In some ways, it is characteristic of the
efforts to use non-sexist language. In this case, the effort
ultimately would be to use "non-age" language.

It may be assumed, therefore, that hearing impaired
older persons experience communication difficulties similar
to those encountered by the younger hearing impaired adult
population. There are variables unique to older persons
which must be considered before such an assumption can be
made. Perhaps the most significant factor is what level of
communication is necessary for the senior citizen to effectively meet his daily needs. The hearing impaired senior
citizen who lives independently, rarely socializing, may not
recognize or even possess any real communicative problems,
maybe due in part to the small amount of interpersonal communication encountered during everyday living. This may be
comparable to some children with hearing impairment.

Greater demands are automatically placed on effective
communication skills for those individuals living in a family
setting. If listening is a struggle, and if asking people
to repeat themselves causes sufficient embarrassment, the
older member of the family may withdraw and retreat, leaving
all discussion and decision making up to the other family
members. Similarly, the senior citizen who resides in an
extended care facility may be unable to effectively deal with
his hearing handicap, thus choosing isolation as a preference
over an uncomfortable interpersonal situation. In addition,
the extended care facility staff and residents, and family
members may not fully understand the implications and frustrations of hearing impairment. Is this any different than
the parent whose child has hearing impairment, the parent who
must learn the ramifications of how hearing loss affects the
child?

Clearly, attention must be directed toward improving
the communication function of older adults with acquired
hearing loss. The same goal applies for children with hearing handicap. With regard to adults, it needs to be indicated that there are those who live in extended care facilities
and others who reside in private residences. A need exists
to assess communication function, directly related to psychological attitude, regardless of place of residence.

Before proceeding directly to communication assessment and its relationship to psychological attitudes, it is appropriate to consider an overall developmental structure. Table 1 depicts this structure.

TABLE 1

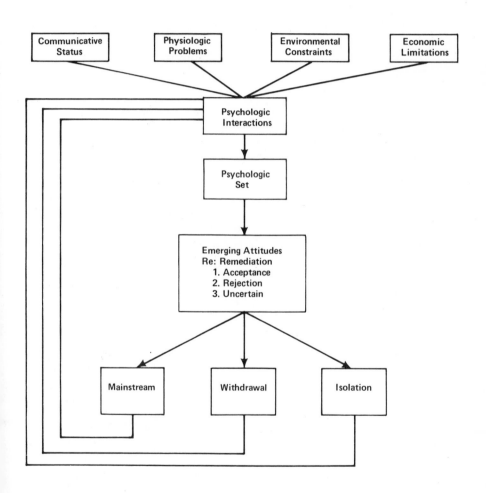

The assumption is made that there are four significant factors which ultimately lead to the emergence of attitudes. These four factors are communicative status, physiologic problems, environmental constraints, and economic limitations. Their collective relevance leads to psychologic interactions which occur in the individual. It is a time of sorting out and processing the impact caused by the four factors; it may be a time of confusion and frustration. These psychologic interactions ultimately will lead to a psychologic set. It is that stage in the structure in which a person begins to develop, if possible, a means by which he can view himself and how he thinks others consider him. As audiologists, we will encounter the attitudes of individuals with regard to the remediation process. The attitude we see, on the part of the client, may be one of either acceptance, rejection, or uncertainty. Our hope is that the client will enter a mainstream in society. He may, however, choose withdrawal or isolation. These latter three aspects probably relate to the psychologic interactions based on the four factors. What has become apparent to this writer is that the audiologist has to be aware of all affecting factors in the rehabilitation process. We do not create the factors found in hearing impaired persons, we inherit them. Although the mission is to remediate, we do not remediate alone because there may be little our efforts can accomplish regarding physiologic problems, environmental constraints, and economic limitations. The attitudes of these adults, therefore, may already be firmly established. If rehabilitation of the so called geriatric client has any potential for success, we will find ourselves working with other professionals and individuals who have some control over the four factors.

Since communicative status, in part, contributes to psychologic interaction, an assessment scale which would subjectively assess the communication function of senior citizens living in health care facilities was developed (Zarnoch and Alpiner, 1977). The scale is referred to as *THE DENVER SCALE OF COMMUNICATION FUNCTION FOR SENIOR CITIZENS LIVING IN RETIREMENT CENTERS* (DSSC). It should be noted that we now regard the name of the scale as inappropriate since it contributes to the labeling of a "minority" group. The DSSC was modeled after the concept of the original *DENVER SCALE OF COMMUNICATION FUNCTION* (Alpiner, et al., 1974). The latter scale was not designed to explore the communication problems of adults living in confined environments. The DSSC, therefore, was designed for this purpose. The persons living in confined environments appeared to exhibit considerably greater difficulty in overcoming their hearing handicaps. This

observation was noted during therapy sessions when comparing
them to adults who were living in self sustaining environments. We further noted that they revealed less interest,
motivation, and concern, not only about their hearing loss
but also what they could do to alleviate some of its detri-
mental effects. We attempted to stimulate their interest and
concern through group therapy sessions. It became apparent
that group therapy was ineffective because we were utilizing
a common therapy plan for all members of the group. The
problem with the group approach was that it did not take into
account an individual's specific problem areas, some of which
related to the other three factors previously discussed.
Thus, the DSSC focused on obtaining specific communicative
status information for planning remediation according to
individual needs.

The DSSC consists of 7 major questions which cover
the following areas of communication: family, emotional,
other persons, general communication, self-concept, group
situations, and rehabilitation. Included under each of the
main questions is a "Probe Effect", and an "Exploration
Effect". The Probe Effect determines the specific problem
areas related to the general question and the Exploration
Effect tries to determine how applicable the general question
is to the individual client. For example (Figure 1.A.),
Question 1 asks, "Do you have any trouble communicating with
your family because of your hearing problem?"

1. *Do you have trouble communicating with your family because of your hearing problem? Yes____ No ____*

PROBE EFFECT I:

a. *Does your family make decisions for you because of your hearing problem? Yes____ No____*

b. *Does your family leave you out of discussions because of your hearing problem? Yes____ No____*

c. *Does your family get angry or annoyed with you because of your hearing problem? Yes____ No____*

FIG. 1.A. *Sample Question with Accompanying Probe Effect Questions.*

The Probe Questions determine if there are specific areas
related to the family which are creating problems for the
individual. The Exploration Questions help determine the
full impact of the problem, if one does exist (Figure 1.B.).
There may not be a family or they may live so far away that
the client never sees them.

EXPLORATION EFFECT

a. *Do you have a family? Yes_____ No_____*

b. *How often does your family visit you?*
    _____

c. *How far away does your family live?*
    In a city_____   Other_____

d. *How often do you visit your family?*
    _____

    *FIG. 1.B. Exploration Effect Accompanying
    Sample Question.*

    _____
    _____

In those cases, the question would be irrelevant and could be
eliminated from future therapy goals. The scale does not
attempt to compare one individual's status with another, but
rather to evaluate the client's impression of his own communication performance.
        Each of the 7 main questions and the 20 probe effect
questions require only a yes or no answer, while the 20
exploration questions may generate client responses other
than yes/no. All of the main questions in the series should
be asked as is, with no manipulation of the phrase. The
Probe and Exploration Effect questions may be manipulated in
order to extract additional valuable information. In that
way, the Probe Effects may act more effectively as a check
on the accuracy of the response to the main question. Exploration Effect questions may be modified as necessary to
identify specific problem areas more precisely. Finally, the
audiologist must review all client responses and make a subjective decision as to whether a communication problem exists
for the individual in each of the 7 major categories.

A sample of the score sheet used to record the client's responses is shown in Figure 2.

CATEGORY	MAIN QUESTION	PROBE EFFECTS	EXPLORATION EFFECTS
	+ −	a b c	a._____
Family	1. ⊏⊐⊏⊐	⊏⊐⊏⊐⊏⊐	b._____
			c._____
			d._____

Problem ⊏⊐   No Problem ⊏⊐

FIG. 2. Sample of Scoring Sheet

For each category appropriate scoring boxes are included for the main questions and probe effects. A + or − is placed in each of the boxes to indicate a response of yes or no. Adjacent to the score boxes is a section for writing the responses to the Exploration Effects. Finally, there are 2 additional boxes for each category, labeled as "Problem" or "No Problem". After examining all of the responses in a particular category, one of the boxes should be checked depending on the audiologist's final decision on whether a problem does or does not exist.

To determine test-retest reliability, we administered the scale twice to 10 different subjects over a 2 week period. The subjects ranged in age from 76 to 94 years, with a mean age of 82. Our intent was to obtain only preliminary reliability data. Table 2 summarizes this information. The summary is only for the main question in each of the main categories. As will be noted, questions 3 and 6 displayed the highest discrepancies, with 4 of 10 subjects (40%) revealing contradictory answers to these questions. The test-retest results for the Probe Effects were similar to those for the main questions. However, it was difficult to determine how reliable the Exploration Effects were, due to the fact that additional comments other than yes or no were required. Overall, it appeared that pre- and post-test responses were in agreement at least 60% of the time.

TABLE 2

Test-Retest Reliability

Results: Reliability Group (N=10)

Questions	Pre- and Post-Test Discrepancies	
1 - Family	3	(30%)
2 - Emotional	2	(20%)
3 - Other Persons	4	(40%)
4 - General Communication	3	(30%)
5 - Self-Concept	1	(10%)
6 - Group Situations	4	(40%)
7 - Rehabilitation	2	(20%)

It should be clear that the DSSC is still in its early stage. At the present time, data on the accuracy of the scale is incomplete, reliability is questionable, and certain problem sections which are ambiguous and/or irrelevant are being revised. Nevertheless, our preliminary investigation of the applicability of the DSSC has provided us with a start in contributing "communicative status" to the three other factors in an effort to develop a psychological model for use with adults. We are convinced that an assessment scale is needed to determine the effects of hearing loss on adults within a more psychological framework.

In essence, our efforts to establish a psychology of hearing impairment for the older adult as related to aural rehabilitation are of recent vintage. We are working at a "grass roots" level in this endeavor. It is this writer's contention that we view the older adult as an adult, preserving the integrity of the individual. Positive psychological attitudes may emerge if the senior citizen realizes that he has not been placed in a category that differentiates him from "normal". The bombardment of semantic terminology stressing deficiencies must be eliminated. We can view the four factors of communicative status, physiologic problems, environmental constraints, and economic limitations in terms of psychologic interactions and attitudes with regard to our aural rehabilitation goals. More important is that all persons can be considered in the same manner, without regard to age. Are we prepared to change our own psychological attitudes?

REFERENCES

1. Alpiner, J. G., Chevrette, W., Glascoe, G., Metz, M. and Olsen, B., The Denver Scale of Communication Function, Unpublished Study, University of Denver, 1974.

2. Alpiner, J. G., Audiologic problems of the aged, *Geriatrics, 18,* 19-26, 1964.

3. Chafee, C. E., Rehabilitation needs of nursing home patients - a report of survey, *Rehab. Lit., 18,* 377-389, 1967.

4. Hull, R. H. and Traynor, R. M., Hearing impairment among aging persons in the health care facility: their diagnosis and rehabilitation, *American Health Care Association Journal, 3,* 14-18, 1977.

5. Kimmel, D. C., Adulthood and Aging, New York: John Wiley and Sons, Inc., 1974.

6. Mead, B., Emotional struggles in adjusting to old age. *Post Grad. Med., 31,* 156-160, 1962.

7. Muskie, E. S., Some perspectives on the problems of
    the elderly, *Hearing & Speech News*, *39*, 3-5, 1971.

8. Myklebust, H. R., <u>The Psychology of Deafness</u>, New York:
    Grune & Stratton, Inc., 1966.

9. Senate Aging Committee launches investigation of
    hearing aids with two days of hearings before
    consumer interest subcommittee. <u>Washington Sounds</u>,
    Washington, D.C.:   (House Publication) 2, July 22,
    1968.

10. U.S. Senate Special Committee on Aging, A pre-White
    House Conference on Aging: Summary of Development
    and Data. Washington, D.C.:   U.S. Government
    Printing Office, 1971.

11. Wolff, K., <u>The Biological, Sociological and Psychological
    Aspects of Aging.</u>, Springfield, Illinois:
    Charles C. Thomas, 1959.

12. Zarnoch, J. M. and Alpiner, J. G., The Denver Scale of
    Communication Function for Senior Citizens Living
    in Retirement Centers, Ch. 8, Rehabilitation of the
    Geriatric Client by J. G. Alpiner (Ed.), <u>Handbook
    of Adult Rehabilitative Audiology,</u> Baltimore: The
    Williams & Wilkins Company, 1978.

Chapter 11

Communication Problems and
Communication Needs in a
Retirement Setting

HERBERT SHORE, ED. D.

As an administrator, I am pleased to join with representatives of many disciplines which collectively have been designated as "helping" professions. Our mutual goal is to see that the added years of life of the older individual are not empty, arid, and frustrating, but rather are characterized by useful purpose and enriched by experiences of self-realization. High on the list of contributors to self-realization is satisfying social interaction, and communication is an integral part of this interaction.

As life goes on we experience a series of opening doors, new opportunities, and expanding horizons. But coupled with this optimistic view of life must be recognition of the fact that life also provides "a whole long series of partial amputations of capacities," (Ross, 1954). Sometimes these are amputations of the capacity to communicate. Some of the aged suffer sudden massive, even total, amputations of what is a uniquely human capacity--language. Wendell Johnson (1961) has written, "There is nothing else about a human being 'more basic' to his humanity than his gift to symbol, the wonder of tongues, the ever-recurring miracle of language and speech". Some older people find this gift seriously impaired or globally snatched away. Psychiatrists, whose clinical tools are largely linguistic, tell us that "disturbances of communication are directly or indirectly responsible for disturbances of behaviors" (Ruesch and Bateson, 1951). The person whose ability to speak or to hear is impaired may be repeatedly frustrated; experience feelings of doubt about his personal worth; become irritable, discouraged, and depressed; and ultimately withdraw from those whose fellowship he needs.

There are indeed some dichotomies which are paradoxical and which require our consideration, if we are to rehabilitate the hearing impaired through non-medical procedures.

On one hand experts state that the level of noise in our society is rising at the rate of one decibel a year and

on the other we are confronted with sound poverty in residences for the aging. It is laudable indeed that this symposium focuses on aural rehabilitation, but this usually
implies our ability to do something to or for the impaired,
when in fact the major contribution we may be able to make is
in learning new communication skills and understanding the
communication environment and relationship.

Perhaps it will be helpful if we define the context
and define some terms. What image is conjured up - when we
refer to a Retirement Setting as a specialized living
arrangement? Are we thinking of vigorous and well aged living independently in Sun City, Arizona? Are we thinking of
those who seek a total environment in an apartment, condo-
minium, town house, retirement village, freed from the daily
chores of meal preparation, light housekeeping, outdoor work?

Is the retirement setting a campus which offers a
continuity of services from independent living to terminal
care? Is it an apartment house, a trailer village, a rest
home, home for aged, nursing home, long term care facility?

Obviously, the setting may be a factor in the kind of
physical and mental functioning and the amount and degree of
pathology found. The greater the psycho-social health services provided the more likely it will be that the population
will be older and sicker.

Entering the geriatric setting, the individual not
only has sensory loss, but also has sound deprivation because
of the nature of the environment. There is a disappearance
or elimination of high sounds, childrens' voices, bird calls,
whistling, singing, the noise experience of the world. We
have the sterile environment epitomized by the "Shhh" of the
hospital, the nurse in white uniform with finger sealing the
lips. The older person has reduced satisfaction from radio,
TV concerts, and this results in further withdrawal, over-
concern with physical function, food, etc.

It has been reported that the incidence of hearing
loss among the institutionalized elderly is even higher than
for the rest of the population. A 1971 survey reported that
1.2 million Americans over 65 live in nursing or retirement
homes; 90 percent of them have significant hearing impairment. In a recent study in Sacramento, California, approximately 84 percent of the nursing home residents surveyed had
significant hearing impairment (McCartney and Alexander,
1976).

In typical health care, a great deal of information
is usually communicated to the patient via hearing. As
Bettinghaus and Bettinghaus (1976) point out,

...the patient is told about medication, is
told when to awaken, when to eat, how to
bathe and many other commonplaces. For the
average patient the system works well. For
the hearing-impaired patient the system may
not work well. Yet few health care facilities
have made formal provisions for alternative
ways of passing along information.

The informed professional should recognize that up to
40% of the aged may have hearing loss, and, in long-term care
units, on the average 80% will have a loss. Thus, health
personnel can always be on the alert to compensate for this
difficulty. This is probably most important in acute care,
since the professional may have only a short time to make
appropriate adjustments for effective communication.
Bettinghaus and Bettinghaus (1976) illustrate the implications in this situation.

The physician, the nurse, the dietician, x-ray
technician, the orderly, and the laboratory
technician may all need to communicate with
any given patient. In a large facility, not
only one physician, but many different physicians may need to communicate with the patient.

When the patient is aged and has a hearing
impairment, a strain may well be placed on the
relationship....The patient who has developed
a long-term relationship with a personal
physician benefits from the physician's knowledge of and adjustment to the disability....
The same patient, when placed in a complex
health care facility, will lose that benefit.
Some of the personnel on the hospital ward
may not realize the patient has a hearing
disability. Other staff who realize the
impairment may not accommodate for it in a
manner that is comfortable for the patient,
and the patient-provider relationship will
deteriorate.

The retirement setting and the long-term care facility are undergoing change. Their traditional roles are being
modified by compelling societal forces which are creating an
array of complex problems. Motivation and purpose may become
obscured and ill-defined. Our ability to perceive need has

outdistanced our ability to provide solutions. We have become aware of the wide spectrum of phenomena requiring clari-
fication and definition. It is imperative that we gain
perspective so that we can structure, in an organized manner,
our observations, experiences and hypotheses, and define our
role, function and objectives more clearly.

The greater number of chronically ill has moved the
aged serving facilities into the health field. The character
of service has taken on new form as it has reflected changing
functions. The medical and para-medical disciplines now per-
meate these settings and merge with their social welfare
aims.

Under such circumstances it becomes readily understandable that we would be motivated to extend our knowledge
about the totality of our residents' needs. The term
"chronic illness" is a mantle which covers a seemingly infin-
ite variety of disorders. As we begin to sort out, identify,
and classify the specific ailments affecting the resident
population, we discover that we are dealing with multi-
disease processes which are frequently, though not necessarily, inter-related. Thus we find an increasing number of
individuals residing in our setting who have been affected
over a long period of time by degenerative processes which
have affected their capacity to cope with their environment.

Regardless of the pathological etiology, sensory impairment creates a problem for the individual in his interaction with the physical environment and in his relationships
with other human beings. The more severe the disability the
more difficult it is for the individual to develop compensatory mechanisms. Weiss (1959) states, "The ability to compensate is limited by the nature, extent, and multiplicity
of impairments." He points out that the individual depends
upon sensory function to obtain information about the environment. He relies upon perception to cope with it.
Freedman (1961) states, "The individual functions in a changing world by virtue of his ability to make predictions about
relationships based on past experience with such relationships. But spatial orientation in the adult organism is con-
tingent upon the integration of a complex assortment of
visual, auditory, and kinesthetic cues." When these processes are interrupted by sensory changes the consequences are
serious. The individual becomes isolated from his fellow
human beings and from his environment, that is, from reality.
There is increasing experimental evidence that such isolation
has severe and massive negative consequences upon the personality structure of the individual. Depression, withdrawal,

anxious behavior, paranoia, and disorientation are some of
the symptoms which appear to be correlated to sensory
deprivation.

The dimension of sensory function must be given a position of prominence in our theoretical formulations if we
are to extend the boundaries of our knowledge.

A universal aspect of aging is sensory loss due to
'normal' degenerative processes. What problems must we take
into consideration when we deal with geriatric care in regard
to cognition and perception? It is these sensory modalities
which are of primary importance in human data processing and
behavior. These aspects of older persons' functioning become
particularly critical as they relate to the matter of placement in a geriatric retirement or institutional setting.

It is a common observation that many who apply for
placement in a protected setting frequently come to us at a
point in life when their resources - physically, emotionally
and culturally, are diminishing or are depleted.

The additional deficits caused by sensory loss tend
to reinforce the dehumanization process which has already
gripped the individual. It becomes understandable why the
applicant places in the lap of the institution the responsibility for taking control over his density. Still there are
life's forces, however, latent, which rebel at this verifica-
tion of his condition. This may in part account for the
trauma we observe on the part of so many new residents.

One of the phenomena that we as health professionals
must guard against is inappropriate diagnosis and inaccurate
labeling. We forget that the retirement facility requires a
great deal of new mapping, that the geography and turf familiar to us can be overwhelming and confusing. If perchance
the individual goes to the left, instead of to the right,
this is not proof of "senility". If the individual's
response is inappropriate it is not necessarily evidence of
mental impairment. As Busse (1967) points out:

> Although vision is important to environmental
> adjustment, hearing seems to be more so. Be-
> cause little has been known of the personality
> effects of the gradual loss of hearing,
> Eisdorfer at the Center for the Study of Aging
> and Human Development at Duke University has
> intensively studied the psychological effects
> of hearing loss on elderly people. It was
> found that a moderate impairment of vision,
> even when uncorrected, has no discernible
> effect on psychological functioning, but

comparable hearing impairment is associated
with significant effects. For instance, to
make an accurate judgment or generalization,
one must recognize stimuli accurately and in
sequence. If an older persons hears A & C,
but not B in a sequence of three sounds, he
has the choice of connecting A & C (thus
making a faulty generalization because B
is not included in his thinking) or of thinking of A & C as separate and reacting as if
they are unrelated. This probably accounts
for some of the irrational thinking we
commonly attribute to senile mentality.

Some years ago I became interested in the growing
body of knowledge about sensory loss and deprivation in the
aged, and as a consequence designed a training program
(Shore, 1976). I found two important things. First, that
though there were important research findings, there was
little attempt to apply the knowledge so that practitioners
could better understand the aged and help them cope, and
second that for the populations I encountered in geriatric
settings had significant hearing loss upon audiological testing approximately one third could be helped by medications,
surgical treatment, or prothetic devices, and the remainder
could not be helped by having things done to or for them.
That taught me that if we were to be truly helpful to the
elderly it was of crucial importance for those attempting to
interact with the aged to improve their communication skills.
Thus in much of the training we do attempt to teach the
following simple rules and steps to all (employees, volunteers, relatives, Board Members, etc.).

- Face the person. Get his/her attention before you start.
  (A hand gently placed on the person's forearm will gain
  their attention). Approaching from behind can startle
  the person.

- Make certain there is good light (so they can get your
  verbal speech read and non verbal body language, face
  expressions, gestures, hand movements, smiles, grins,
  nods, etc.).

- Speak slowly and distinctly. Enunciate clearly the duration of sound aid in processing. There is a loss of
  clarity as well as a loss of volume.

- Ask if you are speaking at the proper volume, but don't shout. Shouting makes one nervous. The listener may be helped and assured if you ask him to repeat the key aspect of a message - did you understand how often to take this medication?

- Very often when we see someone with a hearing aid we raise the level of our voice - this places an additional burden on one who is experiencing aid assisted speech.

- Place in context and give the person a clue. Tell the individual what or whom you are talking about! We are talking about Cousin Louis, or we are talking about Sue's new wig.

- If you repeat use a new key word. Instead of "we bought a new car", you may have to say, "we bought a new Chevrolet" or "a new automobile". Keep sentences short and if you repeat or rephrase make it short and simple.

- Provide a pencil and paper for written communication (especially with the deaf).

- Short frequent contact, a friendly smile, a warm "hi" helps keep the person in contact and lets the person know you are thinking of him as a person.

- Ask direct questions requiring a simple yes or no, rather than those requiring complex answers.

- Single word instructions, e.g. dinner, water, bathroom, may help provide the necessary cuing.

- Don't speak for the person if they are capable of speaking for themselves.

- Do not attempt conversation with the hard of hearing when there is loud background noise, such as a running faucet or blaring TV set.

- Do not talk to the person as if he were an infant and avoid terms such as honey; and don't talk about the person in front of him.

     I have hopefully stressed the need for communication skills in working with the elderly in retirement settings. I believe that the employees want to do a good job and to be

helpful to the residents, but that they are not trained adequately in basic communication skills. Activities and programs and our therapeutic interventions are often less successful than we would like them to be because of the lack of
proper preparation and understanding.

Some years ago I visited a large Catholic Home and
observed a wonderful service. Every Saturday following lunch
the residents knew that there was a prosthetic clinic in the
lobby. One of the Sisters had a manicurist table with all
the necessary equipment to clean and adjust eyeglasses and
hearing aids. She had a fresh supply of batteries, cords and
all the essential items to help the residents "tune in" and
be in touch with their environment. They recognized the importance of helping residents wear their prosthetic devices
and keeping them in good repair.

Our diagnostic formulation, if it is accurate, can
provide us with the cues for treatment of the individual.
The focus on treatment traditionally has been primarily on
the primary degenerative process; use of drugs, of medical
treatments, etc. rather than on the perceptual and sensory
loss. Without giving at least equal attention to the latter
we emphasize the physiological disturbances, which in many
cases are irreversible and represent essentially management
problems. We therefore come to the following conclusions;
our diagnostic evaluations should include (1) a thoroughgoing
appraisal of sensory dysfunction along with the other estimates we make of the person's physiological processes; (2) we
should estimate the degree and quality of behavioral distortion that exists and attempt to differentiate normal charac-
terological manifestations from aberrational ones; (3) an
effort should be made to correlate the physiological findings
(organ damage) with sensory loss; (4) we should begin to
develop concepts of how to help the individual to compensate
for his losses (rehabilitation). This will take into account
spatial organization (architecture), prosthetic appliances,
socially useful roles.

Of particular importance is our need for trained
staff which should have a competence in these specialized
areas. We can look to the theoreticians, researchers and
practitioners in the fields concerned with visual disorder,
auditory loss and perceptual problems, to help guide us. We
must become conscious of the existence of other organized
bodies of knowledge which exist in these fields and become
better informed about these specialities. Rather than seek
to create segregated institutions on the basis of stereotyped
concepts regarding the sensorially handicapped individual we

should attempt to extend our understanding so that such an
individual can live together in the same environment with
other human beings.

The task, therefore, that confronts the institution
is one of freeing itself from smugness, comfort, and laissez-
faire-ism. It must be adventurous in its willingness to
explore new ways of doing things and doing things better.
We must improve and extend our skills in differential diagnosis. We have to acknowledge research and promote an atmosphere in which experimentation is welcome. We do believe
that the institution is a civilizing influence as well as a
therapeutic environment. For the individual it is home and
we are his resource to help him fulfill himself as a social
human being.

Hearing and communication are almost inseparable. We
learn to talk (speech) and to organize what we say (language)
through hearing; we use hearing even when we read, "speaking"
internally the words we read. Few jobs are available today
for the person who cannot hear and communicate with ease;
social activities and friendships become burdensome (if not
impossible) without adequate hearing ability. Those with
normal auditory ability usually fail to understand the problems and consequences of hearing loss.

Normal hearing enables us to communicate; the ability
to hear and understand conversation makes socialization
possible. Golfing, movies, television, dinner parties, lectures and religious functions--all depend on communication to
be satisfying. With poor hearing, one tends to withdraw from
activities and friendships.

In addition to increasing our knowledge of how to
interact and communicate, the context in which that interaction takes place is crucial if we want to meet the communication needs of older people.

Barnlund (1968) and Cassatta (1976) have been helpful
in identifying the essential elements of a therapeutic relationship. These include recognition that such a relationship
is possible when:

-There is a willingness to become involved with older people;
-One or both persons convey positive regard for the other
 person;
-A permissive climate is developed;
-Empathic understanding is communicated;
-The persons are genuine and congruent;
-There is the desire and the capacity to listen.

Egan (1970) summarizes the active process of listening:

> One does not listen with just his ears: he
> listens with his eyes and with his sense of
> touch, he listens by becoming aware of the
> feelings and emotions that arise within him-
> self because of his contact with others (that
> is, his own emotional resonance is another
> "ear"); he listens with his mind, his heart
> and his imagination. He listens to the words
> of others, but he also listens to the messages
> that are buried in the words or encoded in all
> the cues that surround the words. . . he lis-
> tens to the voice, the demeanor, the vocabulary
> and the gestures of the other. . . to the
> context, the verbal messages, the linguistic
> patterns, and the bodily movements of the other.
> He listens to the sounds and to the silences.

Are we really willing to know the individual beyond
his organic or episodic complaint? Do we convey basic
respect or do we control or coerce the other person? Do we
attempt to develop an atmosphere of understanding rather
than one of judging and evaluating the behavior of others?
Are we truly interested, not only in the persons' functioning, but the feelings and meaning of the person's condition?
Can we understand the person's isolation, helplessness, hopelessness, worthlessness?

There is great interest in the provision of quality
of care and quality of life for the aged. Obviously the
quality of life in a retirement setting or elsewhere is related to meeting the total needs of the individual and assur-
ing that the older person has the opportunity for continued
participation and interaction. We can indeed contribute to
life, satisfaction by careful attention to programs of aural
rehabilitation in geriatric settings.

REFERENCES

1. Barnlund, D. C. Interpersonal Communication: survey
    and studies., Houghton Mifflin, Boston, 1968.

2. Bettinghaus, C. O. & Bettinghouse, E. P., Communication
    Considerations in the Health Care of the Aging,
    Aging and Communication, University Park Press,
    129-154, 1976.

3. Busse, Ewald M., Therapeutic Implications of basic research with the Aged, Stoecker Monograph Series No. IV, V. Penn Hospital Phila., 1967.

4. Cassata, Donald M., Communication and the Aged, Perspectives on Aging, 31-35, 1976.

5. Egan, G., Encounter: Group Processes for Interpersonal Growth, Cole Publishing Co., Belmont Colt, 1970.

6. Freedman, Sanford J., Henry V. Grunebaum, Perceptual and Cognitive Changes in Sensory Deprivation, Sensory Deprivation, Harvard University Press, 1961.

7. Johnson, W., Are speech disorders "superficial" or "basic", ASHA, 3, 233-236, 1961.

8. McCartney, James H., A Look at Hearing Loss in Perspective on Aging, Nov/Dec, 10-11, 1977.

9. Ross, M., Some psychiatric aspects of senescence: a review of the literature, Psychiatric Quarterly, 28, 93-112, 1954.

10. Ruesch, J. and Bateson, G., Communication: The Social Matrix of Psychiatry, N.Y. W.W. Norton & Co., 1951.

11. Shore, Herbert, Designing a Training Program for Understanding Sensory Losses in Aging, The Gerontologist, 16, 2, 157-165, 1976.

12. Weiss, Alfred D., Sensory Functions, Handbook of Aging and the Individual, U. of Chicago Press, 1959.

Chapter 12

An Interchange of Ideas

GUEST FACULTY AND AUDIENCE

Cooper: Now is the time for discussion with more
freedom to the questions. The session this morning is simply to make this panel of symposium participants completely
at your disposal for any kind of questions.

Jeanette Fingerman: I have reacted to a statement or
a couple of statements that were made not by the speakers on
the platform, but by two or three gentlemen in the group,
having to do with the use of students in practicum to provide
free services to the community. I just wanted to indicate
that beyond the negative kind of results you might find, we
use students in our community's program as a public relations
job for the profession. The program uses students to provide
testing of elderly individuals at senior citizen service
centers. But we do not jump in and say "your hearing is bad
and we want to test you and do something about it". We start
out by letting them become familiar with us and the students
who are young, attractive, vital, interested and who do a
great selling job. The students have made the thought, indeed, the practice of going to a professional person, much
more palatable. We are able to refer without so much fright,
without so much fear and apprehension on the part of the
older person. We are dispelling some of the myths and some
of the misconceptions. There is one thing we cannot help but
note and that is the condition that occurs when someone re-
tires at the age of 65 and instant poverty is encountered.
Those people still must be served by the profession.

Cooper: I happen to have a few questions. In
Dr. Gaeth's paper it was interesting to note that estimates
of the efficiency of the rehabilitative process were provided. I think it was the naval officer involved who claimed
94% success. That is a very high figure and one of the
things that always confused me about what we are doing and
whether it is any good, is that nobody has reasonable information on how well they are doing with aural rehabilitation
in terms of improved performance for the patient. So this
is a question to the panel, the audience. How good are you
and how do you know that you are that good?

Sue Barris: I am from Los Angeles. I have a 98% success rate and how do I know that? Well, they have paid me for the hearing aid, come back when I recommend they do, and keep buying batteries.

Cooper: Then you judged success on the basis of continued hearing aid use?

Barris: Yes.

Kaplan: I would like to comment on that. I am not so sure that lack of complaint indicates that the person is happy when we are dealing with the elderly population. For some, there is a tendency to simply forget about the hearing aid if it does not work.

Barris: But you ask them, "are you happy"?

Kaplan: Well now, they might be happy or say they are when they come back to you for the first, second, third return visit.

Barris: How about continually?

Kaplan: How continually do you see the people that you sell to?

Barris: At least six times and maybe twenty.

Kaplan: What about after six months?

Barris: Whatever is necessary. I get them after three months, after six months, after nine months if they have a problem.

Kaplan: Okay, but they initiate contact with you if they have a problem. What I am suggesting however is that perhaps the segment of the population we have been talking about does not do that. If they are not happy, they simply put their instruments away and not tell you about the problem.

Barris: In the area where I live, if they had a problem they would tell you very vociferously.

Kaplan: Are you talking about the elderly population?

Barris: Yes, ma'am. I have an office that is in West Hollywood, Los Angeles, California. Demographically, it has the highest concentration of senior citizens or older Americans in the whole world.

Kaplan: That is very interesting and encouraging.

Alpiner: I think the point that John has made is a significant one because he asks the question how do we know we have been successful in therapy? Do we judge our success subjectively on how we feel in a quantitative way, if a client returns or whether they buy a hearing aid? Do we follow what Harriet says in part, that lack of complaint does not mean that people are successful? In some ways it is very disconcerting that the question has to be asked at this

point in the stage of the profession. The implication is
that we have not yet fully developed pre-post measures for
determining our degree of success.

Gretchen Skalbeck: Who is the person who is responsible for this later accountability? I think you have put
your finger on why we do not have appropriate clinical or
research tools to assess the effectiveness of what we do.
The patient has moved along after the aural rehabilitation
program. Unless there is an ongoing study with a university
to bring these people back six months after their treatment,
we never will have this information.

Cooper: Now we have somebody who wants a nice neat
check-off list, performance measure and statistical analysis
to obtain a nice clean judgment of rehabilitation. Yet
there are some individuals who say, my people come back to
me, they claim to be happy, and the question comes up, "Are
you really happy?". Well, at the very least I might concede
without knowing anything about the person, that they are
probably happier than they were. For what reason is an entirely different matter, but you do not come back and spend
money day after day unless you get some sort of benefit even
though it may not be all the benefit that you want. An
interesting way to look at rehabilitation. Can you expect
the private practitioner or the ongoing service clinic (as
opposed to a university setting where presumably research
and furthering of knowledge is an obligation) to do that kind
of statistical analysis? It is a very practical question
because organizations such as CARF expect you to answer it.
They are expecting purely service organizations who want
their accreditation, to come up with statistical information
which demonstrates that they are, in effect, doing a good
job with their rehabilitation technique. That organization
is saying you have got to prove that you are good. So the
question is really not such an innocuous one.

Skalbeck: Now I want to argue on the other side of
this. I did not say anything about checklists, and there are
many kinds of research. If your course is directed to skills
building--speechreading and auditory training, these kinds of
things will lend themselves to one type of follow-up examination. For example: "What did you retain of the skills that
you acquired during the class?" If your orientation to aural
rehabilitation is primarily counseling, improvement of communication dynamics, etc., you need an entirely different
kind of research tool and I am not sure that we have good
tools. There are other professions that counsel people,
psychiatry, psychology, social work, etc., and within the
scope of my reading they do not have tools to measure

benefits from treatment either. If they did have a handle
on it, we could probably be using the same tools that they
are using. But I doubt that they are amenable to T-Tests.

Fingerman: I would like to supplement what has just
been said. In the situation in which we in Cincinnati find
ourselves, we have some idea of our success. In fact, we
have continual and expanded requests for the service where
there was no interest in the beginning from the elderly
themselves. They are now coming to us and saying we would
like to enter your program or have your service.

Cooper: Who is going to set the standards or give
us standards for these sessions? At this point CARF in no
way tells you what you must do to evaluate your program, but
as of 1979, CARF will require demonstration of a program's
effectiveness.

Binnie: I just wanted to make a comment following
Gretchen's comment of a minute ago about accountability, if
that is the word. A few years ago, some of my students and
I were discussing the efficacy of speechreading instruction
as we were involved with it at Purdue, kind of a more traditional approach. We would go ahead and try to do a pre-post
study to see if we could not document all of this toil that
we were putting into the classes and see if it could be reflected in improvement of lipreading ability. To make a
long story short, the pre- and post-test results were the
same. That is, we did not reflect, we were not able to
demonstrate, an improvement in lipreading, at least in terms
of the instrument that we used. However, we included a kind
of questionnaire thing in terms of the approaches, the group
dynamics, the amount of communication skills that the people
gained from this group activity. It was really remarkable
that despite any measured improvement in formal speechreading
skills (this study was written up in Scandanavian Audiology
last year and it is called Attitude Changes in Speech
Reading) there was a tendency at least, to record changes
in attitude, feelings of group dynamics that really were
supportive, indications from significant others that the work
we were doing with the hearing impaired person was being
reflected in his social space. It is tough to document that
kind of thing. Related to Sue Barris' comment that these
people are voting with their feet, you get a feeling for what
is happening when they are saying something positive about
the approach and the significant others with whom they
communicate saying "Hey, things are moving".

Lee Howard: Dr. Kaplan, if I do not overly simplify
what you said, you stated that the person who most appropriately determined the need for rehabilitation therapy was the

client. And you said the person who most appropriately determined how long aural rehabilitation should continue was
the client, is that right?

Kaplan: This is what I have found with the populations that I have been involved with.

Howard: It would seem to follow then that the
person who most appropriately determines the benefit of aural
rehabilitation therapy would be the client. Would you
comment on that?

Kaplan: I agree with you. The kind of framework in
which we are working stresses as its major goal an overall
improvement of communication. I do not feel that I can
measure this in terms of speechreading improvement or improvement on some measure of auditory training. Even if
these measures demonstrated no improvement, it would not
necessarily mean the person was not improving. Therefore, I
feel the most valid way that I as a rehabilitationist can
judge improvement is the report of the client. So I agree
with you completely. The client is the person who is the
best judge of how much benefit he has received when he has
received maximum benefit, and when it is time to quit. It is
not too comfortable. It would be a lot neater if there were
a more objective way to do this, but I think at the present
state of the art, this is the real world.

Alpiner: I would like to ask Harriet Kaplan a question. It is an extension of Mr. Howard's question and I
think it is a two-part question. The first part is how does
the client know that he has a need of help? Number two, how
does a client know what is available to help him after somehow he determines that he needs help?   I think most of us
are familiar with the fact that the general public is not
quite sure about the business of the audiology profession.
I am wondering how senior citizens have become aware of this.

Kaplan: Again, I would like to react in terms of
what we do with our specific population. I am interested in
two things simultaneously. Service to the senior citizen
population and training of students. Since I am interested
in both, I will identify a given senior citizen center from
among the many that exist in our area in terms of the composition of the population and the proximity to the university.
Once I have identified such a place, I will enter it and talk
to the person in charge, whomever that person may be. If he
is receptive, we get ready to set up. We advertise; I will
go in and meet with as many residents as I can get to come
to a meeting, and explain what we are offering. This
includes testing, counseling, classes, etc. At the same time
I will ask the people who run the facility to post

announcements, to repeatedly make announcements in the dining
hall, the one place you can catch them all, and to do this
continually. So we start with those people who are interested. Now why are they interested? Because (1) they recognize they are not communicating as well as they would like
to; (2) they are curious, and we take it from there. Those
who are curious and find after they learn a bit more about
what we are offering that they really do not want what we
are offering, just stop coming. Those who feel it is a benefit continue to come. This is how we get started, and it
grows. It is a very dynamic thing because people are constantly coming in asking to enter the program because their
neighbors tell them about it. This is how we get started.

    <u>Lloyd Graunke</u>: As a relatively naive professional
in this area, I do not have any present ongoing organized
programs. The thought occurs to me that in most cases of
hearing impairment or communication disorders, if you will,
there is no sudden event or onset, no dramatic event, which
says yesterday I heard, today I do not communicate. It is
a gradual process going on by decades, as Bob, I think,
pointed out to us. Therefore, by the time they reach the
age of whatever is considered senior adults, they have adjusted gradually to their society and they may have made
these adjustments to keep themselves satisfied. They may be
in a satisfied mode until the significant others in their
environment indicate that there are problems. Should we not
be taking census of the information or a sensing of the attitudes that the significant others can provide us in setting
up the initial program for these people?

    <u>Garstecki</u>: In the process of starting a new program,
I have contacted senior citizen centers thinking this is a
target group to draw from and indeed most of the referrals
have come through these contacts. However, I am also finding
that our announcements are being passed on to other people
and at the present time I am finding as many referrals coming
from significant others as from the people that I have been
contacting directly.

    <u>Cooper</u>: I have a question for Miriam. Your comments
on the educational process which leads to rehabilitation
audiologist, appeared to be a little critical. What are you
doing to change the education process and what recommendations might you make for any educational system training
individuals to work with the elderly?

    <u>Henoch</u>: I guess my concern, even in my own setting,
is that the emphasis has been on aural rehabilitation for
children rather than adults. Now I am not de-emphasizing
the importance of aural rehabilitation for children.

However, what I am saying is that too many students, in many
of our universities, are not getting the exposure they need
for working effectively with elderly adults. Therefore, they
graduate, go to work, but are not doing this kind of service
because it is a little scary to do something you know very
little about. I think one of the reasons that this has
happened is that some of the educators, the audiologists, do
not know enough about the process of aural rehabilitation
with the elderly to teach it properly. What I am saying is
that we have got to get more of this ongoing work with the
elderly into our programs. I am trying to get this in our
own program with the adult groups that I have started.

One of the problems we have with the program we have
now, is that the elderly adults have to come to us. The
reason we cannot go to them at the present time is that we
just do not have the staff available. We have two and a half
audiologists on our staff and with the extensive supervision
that we do, we are spreading ourselves thin even when we do
the supervision in our own establishment. We have nursing
homes as well as a beautiful senior citizens center here in
Denton, but we cannot convince the people who allocate the
funds that we need additional staff to provide adequate services to these institutions. We cannot afford the loss of
in-house supervision that would result if we sent ourselves
out to supervise students on site at the senior citizen
centers.

Rebecca Haber: I just want to say that my work is
with services for elderly deaf people across the state and I
would like to respond to what you just said, Miriam. One
thing that got our program going and that I would like to
suggest to all of you, and I know that some of you are very
much involved in this already, is the two-way ongoing communication between consumers of the services that you are providing and all your service providers. When there are
limited staff and finances, there are always volunteers. It
is nice to get paid, but many times, especially when you are
dealing with the elderly population, they have a large need
to feel wanted and to feel that they have a valuable function
to the community. I would like to see more ongoing interaction between persons who have already been successful
aurally rehabilitated and the professional staff that continues to provide these services to the elderly community.

Cooper: I am not in a training institution so I kind
of put Miriam on the spot and I would like to put some other
people on the spot. Len, (Lennert Kopra) for two days we
heard about aural rehabilitation for the elderly, but there
are some very, very practical problems in implementing

programs. In an educational situation you do not have eight
to ten hour control over your students. You do not have all
the money and all the staff that is necessary to do the optimum kind of job. How does the University of Texas at Austin
get programs going and accommodate to this particular need--
aural rehabilitation of the elderly?

Kopra: Well, I have had some experience with senior
citizen centers in Austin and have a hearing aid orientation
program for a group of elderly people. Probably the biggest
problem is in getting the people to take advantage of the
service even though it is offered gratis. We screened something like 164 individuals with threshold audiometry in a
quiet room. We thought about recommending that fifty percent
of that group receive complete audiological examination. One
half of the group took us up on it, and of that half, one or
two agreed to attend a hearing aid orientation program. Very
simply, even though the service in our case was handed out on
a silver platter, we could not entice the individuals to the
program. Transportation is frequently a difficulty so we
provided transportation. Those individuals in the community
who do not drive, do not want to come on our campus because
it is very intimidating; we have 40,000 students and it is
like a little city. I do not have a solution, but I think
that we can prove to the public at large that what we do is
indeed good and then develop some of that favorable feedback
that causes others to contact us for service.

Kaplan: John, I would like to react to the question
you asked Miriam. I offer my complete empathy and sympathy.
I have been in exactly the same position, maybe worse. I
have worked as the sole audiologist in the Catholic University program. It is a real problem. The only way that you
can find the time to supervise students in these places is to
cut back on other things. In order to go out to a center for
two hours a week it was necessary to do less clinical work in
our clinic, less personal supervision of ongoing therapy. It
was simply the way I chose to allocate my own time and it was
rough. I think it boils down to money. I think that most of
our universities and colleges today are facing severe budget
crunches and it is going to be difficult to convince administrators to increase personnel. However, if grant money were
available as it is available for model programs involving
children, then we could fund personnel that way. I would
like to see this considered as a possible solution.

Kasten: John, I need to reflect on the response that
Miriam had to your question because I think we have created
a two-pronged problem and we have to address it in that
fashion. In many respects as a professional group we are

caught in a "Catch 22" situation, particularly in training
institutions. It is very true that we are limited in terms
of what we can do and the supervision that can be provided.
Part of what limits us is the fact that we are mandated from
above that we must spend so many hours with each student in
practicum experiences. We are mandated from above regarding
the number of hours each student must spend in practicum experience. As a result, we find ourselves doing the kind of
thing that Jerry referred to. We set up programs in training
institutions not necessarily based upon what people need, but
based upon how many hours the students have to have in order
to get out of the training program and be certifiable. And
then we are faced with not just our favorite audiology type
student, but we are faced with every speech pathologist in
the world in training who needs 15 hours. This is rather a
remarkable figure because it is difficult to tell whether you
can teach anything in 15 hours, or you can teach just enough
to make them dangerous. We are looking at that kind of problem as we try to bring along the people who are going to do
the things that we believe are necessary to be done. Then we
run into additional problems yet. We have not ever, as a
group, faced the problem of this thing we call certification
which everybody feels is important. Audiologists have to be
certified by ASHA and our present organization has done a
good job of convincing people all around the country that the
only good people are the people who have the stamp. Therefore, we have to train people so that they are able to get
the stamp and this has been generally very beneficial. Yet
when we look at certification requirements, we find of all
the things needed for certification, there are only six
academic hours needed in rehabilitation; the thing that we
are supposed to be the expert at. During this past year the
ASHA Committee for Amplification, for example, put in a
recommendation that hearing aid evaluation procedures be included in the certification process. There is nothing in the
certification process that says people have to know something
about hearing aids although almost all actually do. It is
just assumed that if you are an audiologist, you are an
expert. We proposed increasing the number of supervised
clock hours on a graduate level; requiring fifty supervised
rehabilitation hours dealing with amplification systems, and
fifty dealing with the rehabilitation process, not necessarily involving amplification. We were trying to get in the
whole general process of rehabilitation. Then we presented
it to our own committee, the Committee on Amplification, and
to the Committee on Rehabilitative Audiology. The first
thing we heard was, "You cannot do that. If you require that,

we cannot continue to offer a degree because we cannot get
that many hours for our students." The next person said,
"Well, that is great, but we have got to up it. We should
not have just fifty hours, we should have 150 hours of rehabilitation." The Committee on Rehabilitative Audiology almost
beat us with a big stick. I say all this because I think if
we try to evaluate, if we try to find what we are about, how
we do it, if we look at what we are doing in training institutions, we are in big trouble. That is not the place to
look. What do we do in training institutions? We play those
bizarre games to take care of bodies in training, and hopefully, prayerfully, to take care of bodies in need of training. So we have got to go out where the real providers are
and that is where we have to look for our answers and then
hopefully include this in our amplification requirements.

    Cora Martin: I would like to speak to the question
about funding for model projects. The Older Americans Act
provides money for funding model projects. Some of these
monies are disbursed from Washington, others are disbursed
at the state level, but most of them come from your Area
Agency on Aging (AAA). And all of you, if you are interested
in aural rehabilitation, should go and meet the people who
are in your AAA. The United States is divided up geographi-
cally into AAA's so everybody has an AAA. You need to become
acquainted with the people in those agencies and find out
about the kinds of money that they have available for training and model projects because there is a relatively large
amount of money.

    Henoch: I want to say something in addition
to what Cora said about the Area Agency on Aging. I know
that the money is available. When I was in Detroit, the
hearing and speech center I was associated with had quite a
sizeable grant for the aural rehabilitation program. The
grant budget included paying for staff personnel, screening
programs, follow-up audiological examinations, and refurbish-
ing used hearing aids. Each year the money seemed to get a
little greater as we showed them the importance of what we
were doing. So they do know about us and they are very open
to giving you the money if you can show you have a useful and
beneficial service.

    Kaplan: Is this local money or federal money?

    Henoch: The way I understood it, the Area Agency on
Aging received a certain amount of money from the federal government and the Area Agency disbursed it by awarding grants
to various community agencies. A grant committee reviewed
proposals from the various agencies and provided funds

for those projects they felt would be the most beneficial to
the elderly citizen.

Janet Toole: I want to make a comment about the
training of audiology students. I think it is kind of pre-
sumptuous that we are going in to deal with the older population and we do not know anything about them. I do not know
about most programs but I suspect many do not include gerontology courses. Sometimes they give them as allied courses,
but they are not really incorporated and we are not giving
our students the background. I am from Cal State, Los
Angeles, but I have a rehabilitation program for the graduate
students I supervise at the University of Utah.

Cooper: Are you saying that your own educational
program was deficient in a sense?

Toole: Yes, I think I have had as good a background
in rehabilitation audiology as most audiologists have, yet I
did not get anything to deal with the aging. The whole concept of dealing with the older population has to be changed.
Perhaps we can change the way we think of ourselves and the
way we teach our students to think so that we become facili-
tators of maintenance, rather than "fixers". That is, we
should not be going in to measure some level of improvement,
but rather we should be going in to measure maintenance of
an optimum level.

Cooper: Do you mean failure to deteriorate any
further?

Toole: Right. I can see where we could use lay
people in terms of feedback, in terms of working with other
professionals--linking up to a life situation rather than
just working with hearing aids or giving hearing aid orientation or trying to make patients get four more correct on a
discrimination list.

Binnie: I wanted to comment on the training possi-
bilities in various colleges and universities. When I
arrived at Purdue it was obvious that there was not much
going on in terms of aural rehabilitation. Yet with the
knowledge that hearing impairment was the number one chronic
health problem in the United States and with our feeling of
trying to get involved with this population, we did what
Harriet did and I am sure others have done--busted our backs
running around during the week with our audiometers and all
of our materials. We picked up our students and went to this
facility and that facility. We had in mind what we thought
might be some goals in terms of trying to get these various
facilities to pick up, in a year or so, on a contractual
basis, the actual hiring of audiologists on either full or
part time bases. And we have actually been able to establish

that now. We have several off-campus externship possibili-
ties, the Indiana Veteran's Home, American Nursing Home,
Restorative Services and a number of other retirement homes
are available to our students for training. In terms of
Janet's comment, no, we do not have a strong program in terms
of a gerontology program. There are some good courses in
sociology and many of our students take these courses as related area courses. But really, they are learning on the
job, if you will, by virtue of going into that population and
gaining some directed experiences under the supervision of
an audiologist with CCC-A working in those environments.

    Steve Brown: A lot of places I have lived have been
outside the university setting. I was wondering what is being done directly to get Medicare and Medicaid and possibly
insurance companies to recognize hearing impairments; to
finance hearing aids and rehabilitation for people who are in
rural areas. Is there anything being done directly at the
federal level?

    Sue Barris: I can give you some information. We
have the United Auto Workers contract providing for auditory
services for a patient. They will pay for the doctor and
they will pay cost plus a fee for the hearing aid. Many of
our unions, the Retail Clerks Union for example, will pay for
hearing aids.

    Martin: Title XX will pay for a speech and hearing
therapist. I recognize that is different from an audiologist, but they do pay for audiological rehabilitation under
Title XX for people who are eligible for it. It is one of
the few ancillary services that is covered by Title XX.

    Alpiner: I believe that under that Act, the speech
pathologist, not the audiologist, is the one who must do the
aural rehabilitation and it must be prescribed by the physician and must be directly related to some illness or
accident.

    Getting back to Steve's original question; it is my
understanding at this point in time that the services could
be regarded as non-existent or minimal in rural settings.
I tend to agree with the use of lay individuals in a rehabilitation process. There are some things that we have learned
from experience that lay individuals can accomplish, thus
leaving some of the major rehabilitative audiologic aspects
to the audiologist. For those of you who spend considerable
time at extended care facilities of one sort or another, you
realize that sometimes a person wants to talk with you, ex-
press feelings, which can be a very time consuming thing.
However, it is a part of the rehabilitative process; it is
encouraging communication, it might even be the start of the

emergence of the need for communication. As much as an audiologist would like to spend time listening to these people and talking with them, there is not enough time when you consider the numbers of older people needing help. Another aspect in which lay people could be involved, at least I think so, is in the initial screening test for senior citizens to determine whether or not there is a hearing impairment. We also feel that when we use our own scale (Denver Scale) for communication assessment of senior citizens, which is an interview type, that it can be administered by lay people who have been oriented in that process. This relegates significant time for the audiologist to engage in what we might call the problem cases. An analogy is that of the public school speech pathologist who may get bogged down in very fundamental screening which can be done by lay people, volunteers, aides, mothers. The speech pathologist can then spend significant time working in problem areas. I really do not think we should pass up the utilization of lay people but we must clearly define what the limits are.

Binnie: I wanted to quickly respond to the question raised on the availability of aural rehabilitation services outside of the university community. There is a group of nursing homes in the State of Indiana that have hired speech and hearing specialists, audiologists, speech pathologists, who will come into these nursing homes in an intensive itinerant basis. They are licensed audiologists in the State of Indiana and, also, frequently are registered hearing aid dealers; you must have both in our State if you are going to dispense the instrument. They take the responsibility, if you will, for total patient management, including the dispensing and the post fitting services that are necessary in the environment in which the individual resides. It seems to be working quite nicely, at least in some of the rural areas where there are extended care facilities.

Graunke: Since as I indicated I am relatively naive in developing programs, I would like some information. We hear a great deal about the lack of facilities and services out in the non-urban areas and the non-university areas. Has anyone developed an itinerant program that involves a traveling van that is equipped for audiological services and is taken out into rural areas or a non-university setting?

Mark Drum: I mentioned the other day that I worked in a facility like this in middle Tennessee. This is a three year grant program from Vocational Rehabilitation, which is another funding source that is also often overlooked. This particular program was initially designed to go to the Vocational Rehabilitation centers in the very rural parts of

middle Tennessee. I do not know how familiar you are with
the state, but it is the poor people that we were seeking to
help.

We were going into very rural parts of the state and
we served a lot of nursing homes at the same time. At the
time, the program was very effective although I think all of
us that worked on it felt that it was cost prohibitive. It
was incredibly expensive to send a twenty-seven foot van,
with a sound suite and therapy rooms, out to rural areas. I
think that part of the problem was mismanagement in that the
staff was not organized and the trips were overstaffed. I
think that on a limited scale it could be a very viable way
of reaching these people; I think it can work. I believe it
can pay for itself, but it has to be very carefully planned.
We had too much equipment including an enormous van that required a staff of three to go out with it at all times.
Sometimes all three of us would go out and see one client;
other times three of us would go out and see fifty clients.

Henoch: You said you thought it would pay for itself.
Where would these funds come from?

Drum: Third party payments to the university.

Toole: In Utah, the Lion's Club did a lot of vision
screening. That is principally what they are known for.
They have now gone into audiology. They have a van that they
purchased and equipped for audiological services. We have
trained technicians to use the audiometers in the van. After
the screening, they send the audiograms to an audiologist.
The Utah Audiologic Society is a group of audiologists that
we use to interpret the audiograms and then recommendations
are mailed to the individual that was screened. It is a
little too soon to talk about cost effectiveness, but we are
seeing a lot of people.

Deshayes: I would like to make one comment about the
services of service organizations like the Lions. In
Nebraska the Sertoma International Clubs have been very
active in speech and hearing, primarily in hearing. It is
their International Foundation project now and we have started a pilot project with mobile units going out into the
rural areas. Nebraska is primarily rural and I think initially the program is proving to be quite successful. We did
run into a problem. We were buying too much equipment, but,
I think we are changing that around now. It is to the point
that I think it is going to be successful enough that we can
establish satellite centers where we will be able to hire
full time staff. If we need to have further services we can
either go out in mobile teams or refer them to a larger community. But I think it is working out and I think those

service clubs are becoming quite involved; so far they have
never said no when we asked for something. They are willing
to go out and work for these things and I think this is where
we can use the volunteers. Also, in reference to using some
volunteers, they are the people that we can use for motivation, particularly when you have an elderly person in a
nursing home. They can motivate their friends and colleagues
to get into the program, particularly if they are successful
in their rehabilitation. I think it is the same principle as
a laryngectomee going out and talking to a pre-laryngectomee
to tell them what is going to happen; "this is what you are
going to do and you can keep on living".

Cooper: We have gone through some very broad gener-
alizations and some specific comments about the rehabilitative process. If I may take the liberty of focusing on some
more technical kinds of things, I would like to lead out by
asking a question which was submitted for Dr. Kasten. For
the audiologist who does not have electroacoustic analysis
equipment in his particular facility and he is dealing with a
fair number of hearing aids, how can he or she determine if a
hearing aid is at fault due to some sort of specification
discrepancy and when does he know how to send it back and be
sure that some reasonable thing has been done to the hearing
aid. Twelve thousand dollars is a large chunk of money to
have to put out to buy the gear to check the electroacoustic
properties of hearing aids. Is there anything you can help
us with other than that?

Kasten: We are in a spot right now where just a few
years ago it was not necessarily $12,000 it was more like
$28,000 that was needed. Now we are down to the point where
reasonable measurement devices can be purchased for about
$2,500 to $3,000. They are not fully accurate, not by a long
shot and I do not think anybody would say that they really
are. But as far as quick clinical assessment, as far as
being able to get a good picture of the way in which an instrument operates when it is new and the way in which it
continues to operate, they do an excellent job. Now if you
go the next step, one beyond that, and you say that is not
available, then you are back to the thing that most people
are really expert at, but we tend not to pay that much attention to, and that is our assessment of observational data.
We need to pay closer attention to the people that we work
with rather than to the devices that we work with. We can
see a great deal in terms of the individual's ability to perform and staff or friends or family can tell you a great deal
in terms of the way a person performs or does not perform.

A few years ago the Dahlberg Company came out with a little
device that they were selling for $99. It was just a small
box with a series of attenuators in it so that you could turn
the hearing aid on at the level at which it was ordinarily
used, plug it into the device and then you could listen to
the hearing aid in the way in which it was actually worn. The
thing worked like a charm, except after a year the manufacturer quit making it because nobody would buy it. Nobody saw
the necessity for being able to listen to the hearing aid the
way it really worked. I find the little plastic stethoscope
that you can get from most hearing aid dispensing suppliers
for about four dollars is an excellent device to enable you
to listen to hearing aids in the manner in which they are
typically worn. To address the question of knowing if the
problem with the hearing aid has been effectively handled by
the repair facility, I can only tell you what we have found
to be successful. We tell people to request written verifi-
cation of the repair that has been completed. This tends to
be fairly effective in terms of documenting modifications or
repairs actually carried out.

Cooper: Other comments to the question of whether or
not a hearing aid is working when you do not have the equipment to check it out. How do you solve your problem?

Audience: Well hopefully by your sound field evaluation you will be able to come up with some indication that
the person is doing as well as you would expect him to. If he
is not, then you have to either assume that the hearing aid
is broken, or distorting, or malfunctioning in some other way,
or the person's hearing has changed. That may not be a very
good indicator, but in the absence of anything else it will
provide some information.

Kasten: Well, if I could talk from the other side,
one of the big problems that the repair facilities face is the
number of instruments that go back with the notation, "does
not work right" and they are supposed to fix it with only that
limited information. Part of the time it is the fault of all
of us because we tell a patient, "Well, your hearing aid is
certainly not working right, it needs to be repaired". So
the patient fixes it himself or he takes it back to where
he bought it and the dispensor sends it in to the repair
facility for them with just the comment, "does not work
right". Then the aid is returned and the patient comes back
and says "it still does not work right" and we complain to
the factory because they did not fix what was wrong. This is
not a criticism in any way, since the people who are in repair facilities are genuinely, honestly trying to do the best
job that they can. Most of them who are involved in the

process of repair or who are involved in the process of con-
struction, really do not know anything about the use of
hearing aids. They know how to build them, they know how to
fix them, they know how to open them up and see that everything is where it should be and see to it that the circuits
are properly connected and things are functioning appropriately. Beyond that however, they are not trained to try to
determine, out of a myriad of characteristics, and a myriad
of possible malfunctions, what might be the key factor that
makes this one malfunction. It is a sizeable problem and the
more rural you go in the United States, the bigger the
problem gets.

Cooper: Bob (McCroskey), I think the implications
of your paper were rather clear with respect to rate of
speech. Given an elderly individual with some fusion distortions or inadequacies, what is the implication for aural
rehabilitation?

McCroskey: Yesterday a young lady rose and said that
she discovered she could understand better when the speaker
was not talking through the PA system and she was getting the
information through a hearing aid. I suspect that there was
some very small time discrepancy between the live voice arri-
val time that she was getting on a direct line from the
speaker, and the electronic signal that was coming from a
still greater distance from above. In addition to that, a
portion of the signal was coming off the hard surfaces of the
proscenium arch. What we have is a setting where there are
too many signals. This may provide acoustic filler for some
of the pause-times that we normally require in making certain
kinds of distinctions--not just phonemic distinctions, but
patterns, also. I guess you can infer that if you are going
to do some aural rehabilitation, then you had better know
some of the acoustic characteristics of the room in which you
are going to do it, or it becomes a self-defeating situation.
I discovered after our meeting yesterday that there are certain spots in this room where people cannot distinguish the
fact that there are two tone pulses when the two tone pulses
are 40 milliseconds apart--normally, a very easy listening
task for the ear. And again, we have some spots where the
distance from the tape recorder to listeners' ears introduce
certain time delays, that interact with the reverberant characteristics of the auditorium to mask out the silent interval
between the two tone pulses.

Audience: In terms of providing rehabilitative services for older people we deal with their self-image. I have
seen it come up in the literature. Do you feel that we can
write goals appropriately for self-image work and if so what

are some specific techniques that could be used? Will the
psychologist start becoming uptight about our working with
this aspect of rehabilitation?

    McCroskey: Self-image is the result of an individ-
ual's notion of how he has coped. If one sets up situations
where he infers from what he has done that he has coped, then
his self-image shifts.

    Audience: So your behavioral objective would be,
"He will be able to cope?"

    McCroskey: Indeed, as long as the tasks are within
the range of capability. The individual can infer from
little success over time that he is coping and this shifts
the image.

    Alpiner: I think that self-image deals with the
reality of the situation--that point in time where the individual happens to be. As much as I like behavioral objectives, I am not sure that I would be able to write them for
this population. What haunts me and what I attempted to
state yesterday, was that the older person is not totally
responsible for his self-image or his reality, or the way he
feels, because it is those people in the individual's environment who have already labeled that individual in a
variety of ways. I think there is a spinoff from the way
those of us in the environment label the individual. It is
like the senior citizen has inherited the self-image inappro-
priately from most people in the environment who have
attached false labels for him. I guess that is my new bias.
I want to avoid labeling. I would very much like to get
away from the terms "aged" and "elderly" and "older" because
they denote very negative concepts. It cannot help but be a
spinoff for the self-image.

    McCroskey: May I pick up on that a little bit? I
think we are really together, Jerry. You are saying the
environment imposes the self-concept, partially at least.
And I am saying the individual infers his self-concept from
what he experiences with the environment. Now let me illustrate it a little bit. If the individual attempts to communicate in social settings where the room characteristics
are bad, and he has difficulty understanding the speakers,
and the background noise is such that he is having trouble
with pulling the signal out of it, then he infers that he is
socially inept. If an individual is in a setting where his
ability to follow verbal instructions is beginning to slow
down, those with whom he is interacting will infer that he is
not able to handle the setting. Now, one can provide situations for the elderly person where the listening is easier
and the signals can be processed better. Then the elderly

person will begin to infer that he is handling the world he
is in, instead of feeling that he is losing his grasp of it.

Alpiner: I do not disagree with what you say, from
what I would regard as somewhat of a very limited speech and
hearing viewpoint. I think that all of us tend toward this
narrow view from time to time. Your emphasis was on one
aspect of communication but I want to look at the individual
in terms of the total impact in that environment, the self-
image of that individual in regard to his total feelings.
The approach you take, in my own opinion, is that in remediation of the senior citizen, the emphasis is going to be on
straight communication hearing therapy. That does not take
into account the great dynamic of the human being. Maybe the
person is having difficulty in a communication situation, and
it is quite correct that we should look at how we might improve the situation, but that does not negate part of the
psychological interactions that might have occurred. That
person may already have developed the symptoms of withdrawal
or isolation, or perhaps of inferiority; dealing only with
the communication problem does not alleviate the problems
which have already been extended for the individual.

Cooper: I would like to say something. There are
two aspects of what these two gentlemen are talking about.
I see Jerry talking about that which is imposed by society
and I see Bob talking about that which the individual thinks
of himself, relatively independent of what society thinks.
I think the difference between the two is something which you
really have to take into account.

I happen to know a teenager, who for one reason or
another, ended up at the Marine Military Academy in
Harlingen, Texas. That means a crew cut and a military
uniform, with no civilian clothes for extended periods of
time. That also means living in a community where there are
no other military bases and that is the only uniform that is
seen. You have a context where all the kids are wearing
long hair and "you guys look funny"; I think that is what
Jerry is accenting. Then there is a group of individuals
within the Marine Corp Academy who over many hours a day,
try to tell the kids, "you are better than they are, they are
the crazy ones, you are the only sane ones". They build in
some of those kids enough internal image, enough satisfaction
with that internal image, that what the kids do when they get
out into the street does not matter because they do not care
about the civilians. You are dealing with the kind of information that Roger presented yesterday, "put on a hearing aid
and people will think you are dumb". It may happen to any
one of us and we have concrete information that people are

going to be looking at us funny. How do you save yourself
from that? You save yourself from that because of your own
internal respect which may or may not go along with what
society thinks. I am suggesting to you that you can tell
your patients, "hey, you are okay, and those other people are
really nuts". I think the therapists can address themselves
to this self-image and mold it through careful listening
situations--can do it explicitly. "You are going to go out
there with a hearing aid and people are going to laugh at
you. Just let them laugh, because you are okay and you can
stand up under it!" I think this is a part of what we can do
in the overall context of rehabilitation and it just suddenly
came to me that these two gentlemen are really talking about
two aspects of the same thing and two dominant kinds of influence that are applied.

Martin: I would like to talk a little bit from the
gerontologists' point of view. There is a national study
conducted by the Gallup organization which looks at attitudes
toward aging. The thing that is most astonishing, at least
most astonishing to us, is that older people share all the
myths and sterotypes about aging of those of us who are
younger. For example, they are not sure that older people
should have sexual relations. They feel that older people
are lonely and isolated; therefore, I do not think we are
going to be able to train everybody not to use labels that
differentiate us. I think we are going to call children,
children, and adolescents, adolescents, and older people,
older people. It seems to me that the thing we have got to
do is educate everybody--ourselves and everyone else, to
think that old is beautiful. Rather than changing the labels,
I would like to see the label become a badge of honor.

Index